THE
DIABETES
HANDBOOK

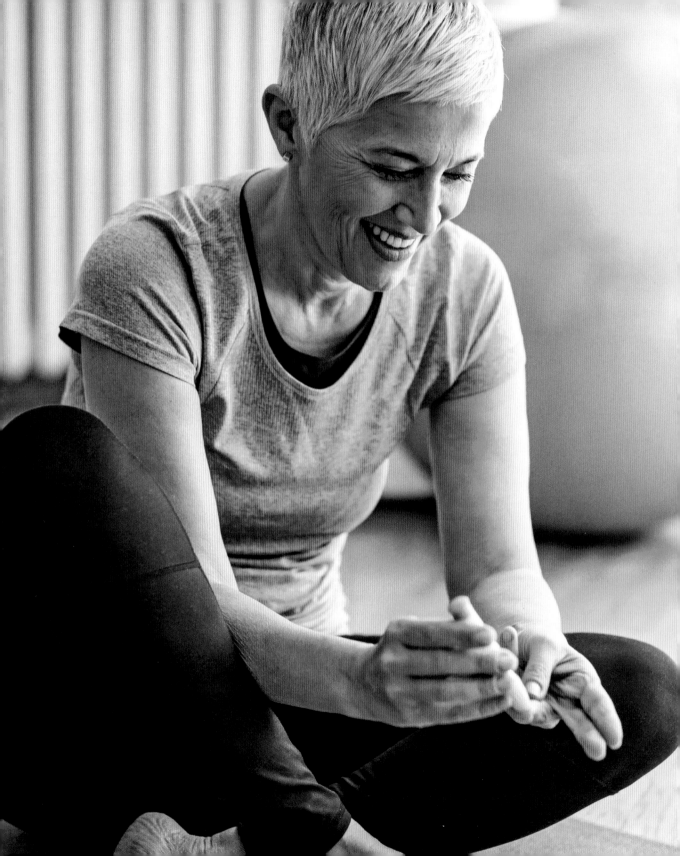

THE DIABETES HANDBOOK

Rosemary Walker

Contents

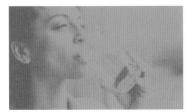

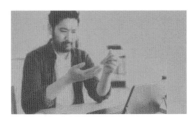

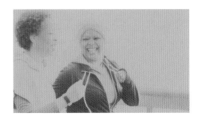

What is diabetes?

Managing your blood glucose

Eating, drinking, and being active

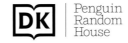

Penguin Random House

DK LONDON

Project Art Editor
Steve Woosnam-Savage

Production Editor
Gillian Reid

Senior Production Controller
Meskerem Berhane

Managing Art Editor
Michael Duffy

Jacket Design Development Manager
Sophia MTT

Lead Senior Editor
Martyn Page

Senior Editors
Rob Houston, Janet Mohun

Managing Editor
Angeles Gavira Guerrero

Associate Publishing Director
Liz Wheeler

Publishing Director
Jonathan Metcalf

Art Director
Karen Self

DK INDIA

Lead Project Art Editor
Anjali Sachar

Project Art Editor
Meenal Goel

Assistant Art Editors
Garima Agarwal, Arshti Narang

Managing Art Editor
Sudakshina Basu

DTP Designers
Ashok Kumar, Bimlesh Tiwary

Pre-production Manager
Balwant Singh

Senior Editor
Suefa Lee

Senior Managing Editor
Rohan Sinha

Senior Jacket Designer
Suhita Dharamjit

Senior Picture Researcher
Surya Sankash Sarangi

Picture Research Manager
Taiyaba Khatoon

Production Manager
Pankaj Sharma

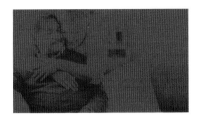

Living with diabetes

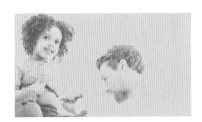

Children and young people

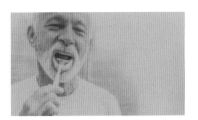

Dealing with complications

* Some topics in the book are marked with an asterisk. This indicates that specific local information about the topic can be found in Notes (p.202).

First published in Great Britain in 2020
by Dorling Kindersley Limited
DK, One Embassy Gardens, 8 Viaduct Gardens, London SW11 7BW

Text copyright © Rosemary Walker 2020

Copyright © 2020 Dorling Kindersley Limited

A Penguin Random House Company

Rosemary Walker has asserted her right to be identified as the author of this work.

10 9 8 7 6 5 4 3 2 1
001–315211–Nov/2020

All rights reserved.
No part of this publication may be reproduced, stored in or introduced into a retrieval system, or transmitted, in any form, or by any means (electronic, mechanical, photocopying, recording, or otherwise), without the prior written permission of the copyright owner.

A CIP catalogue record for this book is available from the British Library.
ISBN: 978-0-2413-9326-0

Printed in China

For the curious
www.dk.com

Medical consultant
Graham Toms, Honorary Consultant Physician and Endocrinologist at Barts Health NHS Trust

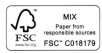

MIX
Paper from responsible sources
FSC™ C018179

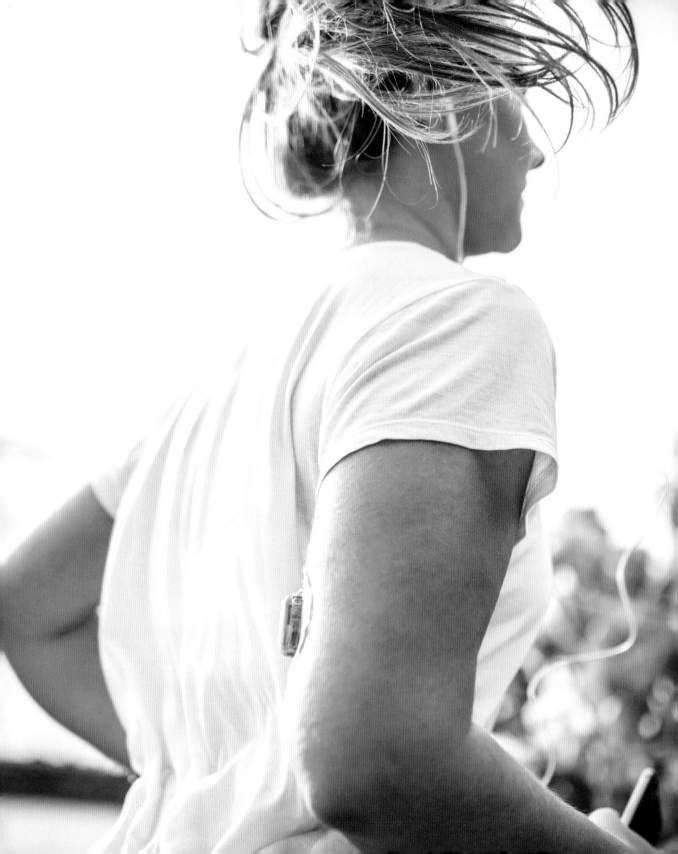

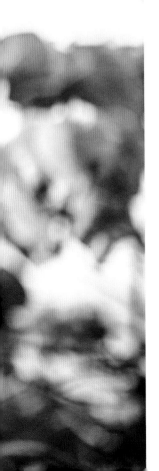

Foreword

You are the expert in your own life. That is my firm belief that lies at the heart of this book. You can make decisions and choices that are right for you, supported by reliable diabetes resources, and empathic, non-judgemental health professionals, who contribute their expertise in diabetes as a health condition.

Diabetes is not a "one size fits all" condition. Every individual experiences it differently, and there are various ways in which it can be treated and managed. In turn, the wider world of diabetes is continually revealing new research evidence and developing new technology to make managing the condition easier and more compatible with your everyday life. Particular attention is also being directed towards finding ways of preventing and curing diabetes, which are our ideal goals. I have tried to make this book reflect all of this, and to give you hope and reassurance.

Among the most important aspects of living with diabetes, the support and society of others who are also experiencing it can be an enormous help in coping with the practical burdens it brings and in staying or becoming emotionally healthy. Throughout these pages, I have tried to encourage everyone who wishes to, to seek out the many opportunities available today to meet, share, and compare with others who live with diabetes. It can be a huge relief to know that you are not alone.

I wish you every success as you start or continue to live with diabetes.

Rosemary Walker

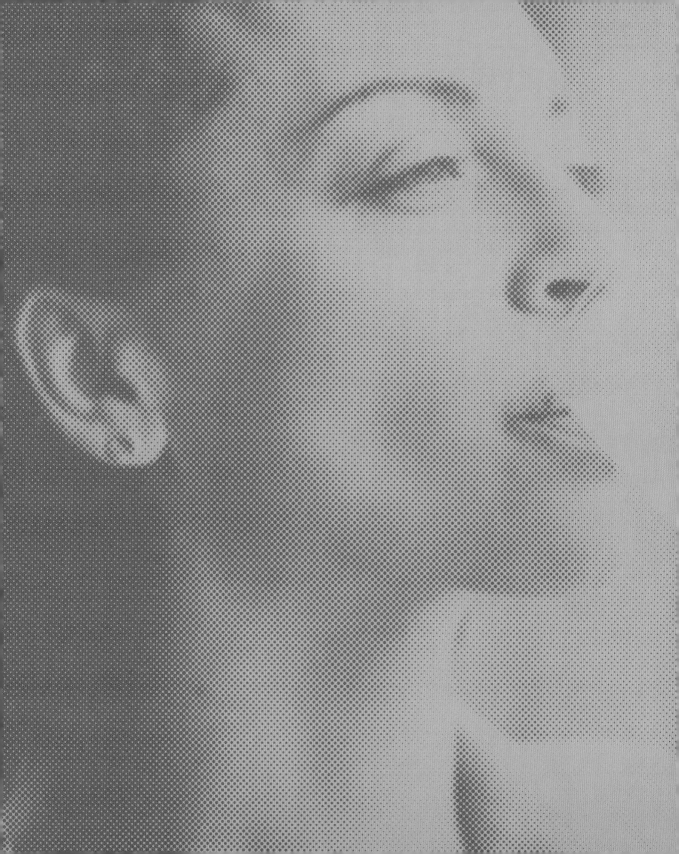

What is diabetes?

Understanding diabetes

All your body cells need energy. Their primary source is glucose, which needs the hormone insulin in order to enter the cells. In diabetes, there is a lack of insulin or insulin cannot do its job properly, which causes various symptoms and health problems.

What is diabetes?

In diabetes, glucose in the blood cannot get into your body cells and so they are deprived of their usual source of energy. Your body tries to remove excess glucose in the blood by excreting it in urine, and it uses fat and protein (from muscle) as alternative energy sources. This disrupts your body processes and leads to the symptoms of diabetes (see pp.18–19).

How the body usually uses glucose

When you eat carbohydrates, they are broken down into glucose, which passes from the digestive tract into the bloodstream and from there into body cells, where it is used to provide energy. Some glucose is also stored in the liver and muscles in the form of glycogen.The level of glucose in the blood is controlled by two main hormones: insulin and glucagon. These work together to keep your blood glucose level within a narrow range. Both hormones are produced in the pancreas, by clusters of cells called the islets of Langerhans. There is a constant background level of insulin but when your blood glucose rises, extra

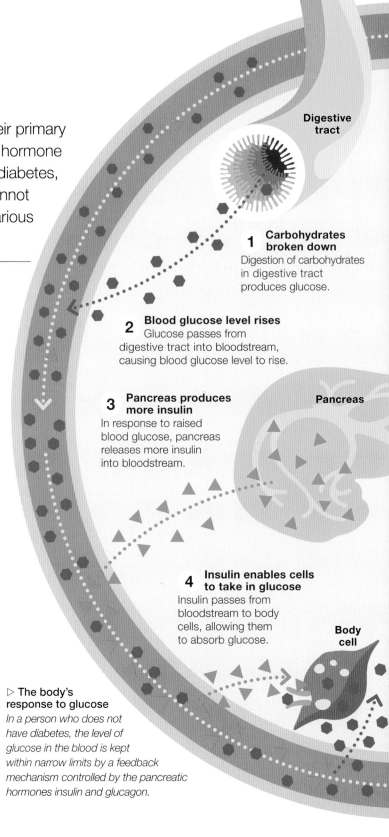

Digestive tract

1 Carbohydrates broken down
Digestion of carbohydrates in digestive tract produces glucose.

2 Blood glucose level rises
Glucose passes from digestive tract into bloodstream, causing blood glucose level to rise.

3 Pancreas produces more insulin
In response to raised blood glucose, pancreas releases more insulin into bloodstream.

Pancreas

4 Insulin enables cells to take in glucose
Insulin passes from bloodstream to body cells, allowing them to absorb glucose.

Body cell

▷ **The body's response to glucose**
In a person who does not have diabetes, the level of glucose in the blood is kept within narrow limits by a feedback mechanism controlled by the pancreatic hormones insulin and glucagon.

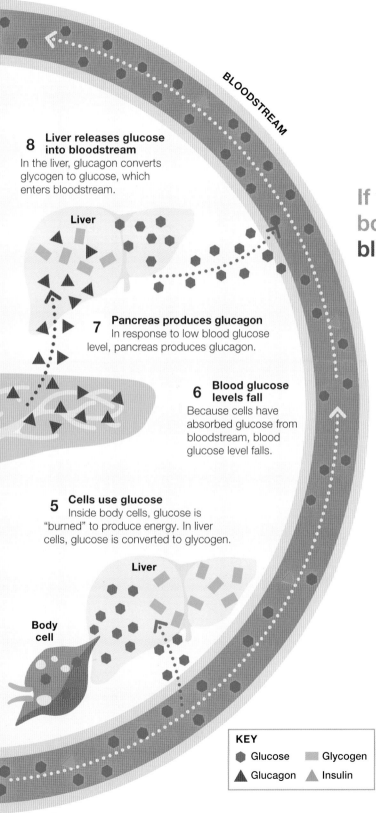

8 Liver releases glucose into bloodstream
In the liver, glucagon converts glycogen to glucose, which enters bloodstream.

Liver

BLOODSTREAM

7 Pancreas produces glucagon
In response to low blood glucose level, pancreas produces glucagon.

6 Blood glucose levels fall
Because cells have absorbed glucose from bloodstream, blood glucose level falls.

5 Cells use glucose
Inside body cells, glucose is "burned" to produce energy. In liver cells, glucose is converted to glycogen.

Liver

Body cell

KEY

⬡ Glucose   ▬ Glycogen

▲ Glucagon   ▲ Insulin

insulin is released. Insulin acts like a key, unlocking body cells so that glucose can enter. When your blood glucose falls, your pancreas releases more glucagon, which converts glycogen in your liver back to glucose. This enters your bloodstream and blood glucose rises again.

If you have **diabetes,** your body **cannot control** your **blood glucose** effectively

What is different in diabetes?

When you have diabetes, you do not produce any insulin, produce too little of it, or your body cells are resistant to its effects. As a result, glucose builds up in the blood and causes symptoms such as passing large amounts of urine, due to your body removing the excess glucose by filtering it out into the urine. Because your body cannot use glucose for energy, it uses its muscle and fat stores instead, which can cause symptoms such as weight loss. A blood glucose level that is only slightly raised – a condition known as prediabetes or borderline diabetes – may not produce symptoms and may be detected only by a blood test (see pp.20–21). A blood glucose level that is significantly above the usual range indicates diabetes.

Types of diabetes

Although diabetes is often referred to as if it were a single condition, there are actually different types. The main ones are type 1 (see pp.12–13) and type 2 (see pp.14–15) but there are also other types (see pp.16–17), such as gestational diabetes and maturity onset diabetes of the young, or MODY.

Type 1 diabetes

In this type of diabetes, your pancreas does not produce any insulin. As a result, your body cells cannot absorb glucose, your blood glucose level rises unchecked, and your cells are deprived of their primary energy source, leading to symptoms such as fatigue, passing large amounts of urine, and weight loss.

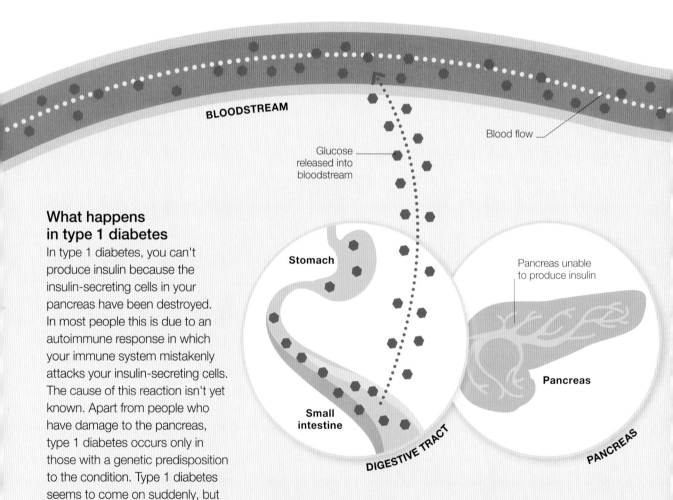

BLOODSTREAM

Blood flow

Glucose released into bloodstream

Stomach

Small intestine

DIGESTIVE TRACT

Pancreas unable to produce insulin

Pancreas

PANCREAS

What happens in type 1 diabetes

In type 1 diabetes, you can't produce insulin because the insulin-secreting cells in your pancreas have been destroyed. In most people this is due to an autoimmune response in which your immune system mistakenly attacks your insulin-secreting cells. The cause of this reaction isn't yet known. Apart from people who have damage to the pancreas, type 1 diabetes occurs only in those with a genetic predisposition to the condition. Type 1 diabetes seems to come on suddenly, but destruction of the insulin-secreting cells can start months or years earlier, and it is not until about 80 per cent or more of these cells have been destroyed that symptoms typically appear.

1 Glucose enters blood
During digestion, glucose is released from the digestive tract into the blood. Normally, this triggers mechanisms to absorb the glucose – including the release of insulin by the pancreas – which lower the blood glucose level.

2 No insulin available
In type 1 diabetes, the insulin-producing cells of the pancreas have been destroyed, so no insulin is released. Insulin "unlocks" body cells, allowing them to absorb glucose from the blood. Without insulin, the blood glucose level remains high.

FEATURES OF TYPE 1 DIABETES

- Can develop at any age, although it is less common for the condition to develop after the age of 40

- Body doesn't produce any of its own insulin

- Symptoms usually come on quickly

- Needs lifelong treatment with insulin, administered by injection or a pump

- It is an autoimmune condition, independent of body weight

- Cannot yet be prevented or reversed

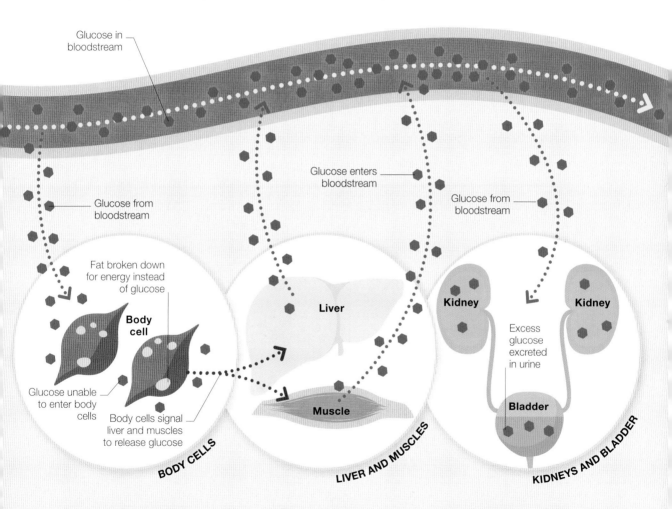

Glucose in bloodstream

Glucose enters bloodstream

Glucose from bloodstream

Glucose from bloodstream

Fat broken down for energy instead of glucose

Body cell

Liver

Kidney

Kidney

Excess glucose excreted in urine

Glucose unable to enter body cells

Body cells signal liver and muscles to release glucose

Muscle

Bladder

BODY CELLS

LIVER AND MUSCLES

KIDNEYS AND BLADDER

3 Cells starved of glucose
Because the body cells cannot absorb glucose from the blood, they are deprived of their primary source of energy. However, they still need energy to function, so they break down fat as an alternative energy source.

4 Blood glucose continues to rise
Starved of glucose, body cells signal the liver and muscles to release more glucose into the blood. However, without insulin, this extra glucose cannot enter the cells and so the blood glucose level rises further.

5 Kidneys produce more urine
To remove excess glucose from the blood and attempt to reduce the blood glucose level to normal, the kidneys filter out the excess glucose, producing large amounts of glucose-containing urine.

Type 2 diabetes

In type 2 diabetes – the most common form of the condition – your pancreas produces some insulin, but either in insufficient amounts and/or your body cells are resistant to its action. As a result, your cells receive too little glucose and your blood glucose level rises too high.

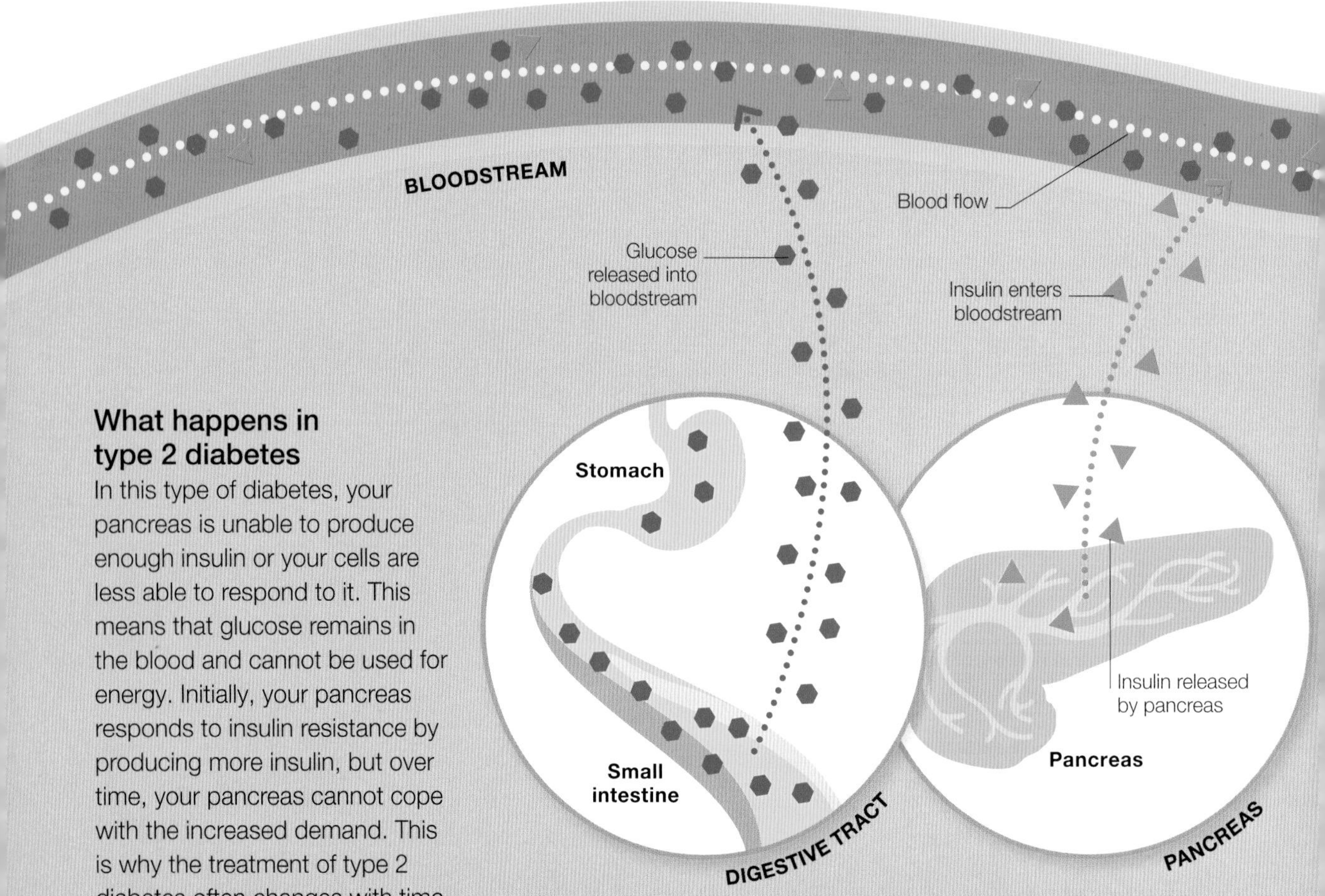

BLOODSTREAM

Glucose released into bloodstream

Blood flow

Insulin enters bloodstream

What happens in type 2 diabetes

In this type of diabetes, your pancreas is unable to produce enough insulin or your cells are less able to respond to it. This means that glucose remains in the blood and cannot be used for energy. Initially, your pancreas responds to insulin resistance by producing more insulin, but over time, your pancreas cannot cope with the increased demand. This is why the treatment of type 2 diabetes often changes with time and eventually you are likely to need insulin. Type 2 diabetes is often, although not always, associated with being overweight, and also with the accumulation of fat deposits around the liver and pancreas.

Stomach

Small intestine

DIGESTIVE TRACT

Insulin released by pancreas

Pancreas

PANCREAS

1 Glucose enters blood
During digestion of food in the digestive tract, glucose is produced by the breakdown of carbohydrates. This glucose then passes through the wall of the intestine into the bloodstream, which circulates it to all parts of the body.

2 Insulin produced
On detecting glucose in the blood, the pancreas releases extra insulin. This hormone is essential to enable body cells to take in glucose, but in type 2 diabetes, the pancreas produces too little insulin or the body cells are resistant to it.

FEATURES OF TYPE 2 DIABETES

- Usually starts in later adulthood, but becoming more common in teenagers and young adults

- Body produces insulin but either too little and/or the body cells are resistant to its action

- Symptoms may come on gradually or may not be obvious

- Managed with healthy eating, physical activity, medication, and sometimes insulin. Treatment may change over time

- Affected people are often overweight

- Losing weight and reducing fat stored around the liver and pancreas may produce a remission

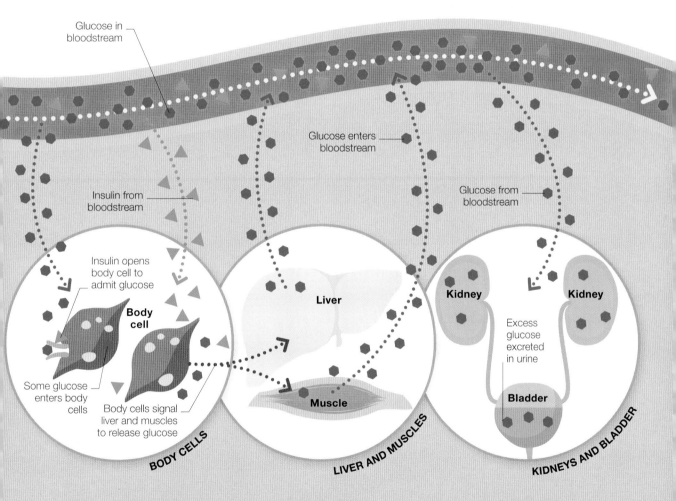

Glucose in bloodstream

Glucose enters bloodstream

Glucose from bloodstream

Insulin from bloodstream

Insulin opens body cell to admit glucose

Body cell

Liver

Kidney   **Kidney**

Excess glucose excreted in urine

Some glucose enters body cells

Body cells signal liver and muscles to release glucose

Muscle

Bladder

BODY CELLS

LIVER AND MUSCLES

KIDNEYS AND BLADDER

3 **Cells starved of glucose**
Due to the lack of insulin or the inability of the body cells to utilize it fully, the cells can take in only a small amount of glucose. As a result, they cannot obtain as much glucose as they need for their energy requirements.

4 **Glucose rises further**
To try to get more glucose, the body cells signal the liver and muscles to release glucose into the blood. However, most of this glucose cannot enter the cells and remains in the blood, causing the blood glucose level to increase even further.

5 **Kidneys produce more urine**
As in type 1 diabetes, to try to reduce the blood glucose to normal, the kidneys filter out the excess glucose from the blood, producing large amounts of glucose-containing urine as a result.

What happens in gestational diabetes

Diabetes that develops during pregnancy is mainly due to placental hormones reducing the effectiveness of insulin, combined with the pancreas not being able to produce enough extra insulin to compensate. As a result, body cells cannot take in enough glucose to reduce the raised blood glucose level.

Other types of diabetes

In addition to the familiar type 1 and type 2 diabetes, there are other types. Diabetes may also occur as a result of another medical condition or treatment; this is known as secondary diabetes.

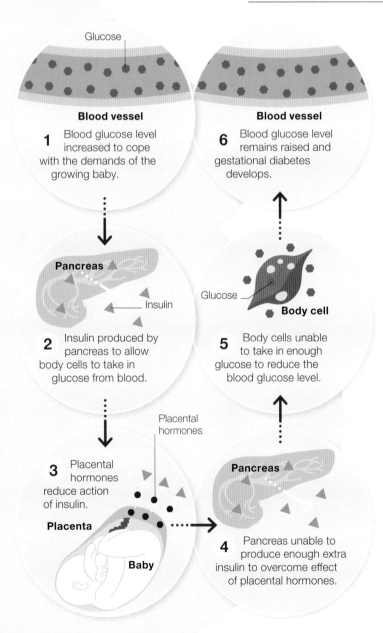

Glucose

Blood vessel

1 Blood glucose level increased to cope with the demands of the growing baby.

Blood vessel

6 Blood glucose level remains raised and gestational diabetes develops.

Pancreas

Insulin

Glucose

Body cell

2 Insulin produced by pancreas to allow body cells to take in glucose from blood.

5 Body cells unable to take in enough glucose to reduce the blood glucose level.

Placental hormones

3 Placental hormones reduce action of insulin.

Placenta

Baby

Pancreas

4 Pancreas unable to produce enough extra insulin to overcome effect of placental hormones.

Gestational diabetes

Diabetes that first appears in pregnancy is known as gestational diabetes. Sometimes, it is type 1 or type 2 diabetes that was not diagnosed before pregnancy. More often, however, it first appears during pregnancy, at around 24–28 weeks, and disappears when the baby is born. Women who develop this type of diabetes are at high risk of getting gestational diabetes again in future pregnancies and also of developing permanent type 2 diabetes within a few years. When you are pregnant, your body increases its blood glucose to cope with the demands of a growing baby and more insulin is needed. However, the hormones produced by your placenta make insulin less effective. If your insulin production isn't able to overcome this reduced effectiveness, glucose remains in the blood and gestational diabetes develops. This condition may not cause symptoms, but it will be detected during routine antenatal checks. If you do develop gestational diabetes, you will be offered personalized treatment and care during your pregnancy (see pp.136–137).

Maturity onset diabetes of the young

Commonly known as MODY, this is a rare type of genetic diabetes that occurs in people under 25 who have a family history of diabetes in at least two generations. MODY is often inadvertently diagnosed as type 1 or type 2 diabetes. In addition, MODY is often treated with insulin when in many people it could be managed successfully with other diabetes medications or, in some people, without any medication.

Latent autoimmune diabetes in adults

This condition (often called simply LADA) has features of both type 1 and type 2 diabetes and so is sometimes referred to as "type one-and-a-half diabetes". LADA typically develops from your 30s onwards. Like type 1, it occurs because your pancreas stops producing insulin, thought to be due to the immune system attacking your insulin-producing cells. However, unlike type 1, your insulin-producing cells continue to produce some insulin for months or even years. The symptoms of LADA are typical of diabetes and tend to come gradually: persistent tiredness; excessive urination; continual thirst; and weight loss. If you are suspected of having LADA, treatment will be with tablets and/or insulin, depending on your blood glucose levels.

Neonatal diabetes

This type of diabetes is extremely rare and is defined as diabetes diagnosed before the age of 6 months. It is caused by a genetic mutation that affects insulin production. There are two types of the condition: temporary and permanent. In the temporary type, the condition typically disappears by the age of about 12 months. The permanent type is lifelong and can be confirmed by genetic testing. Treatment may be with tablets or insulin.

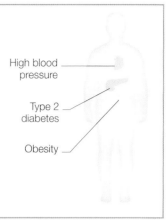

METABOLIC SYNDROME
This condition is not strictly a type of diabetes but is an umbrella term for the combination of high blood pressure, obesity, and type 2 diabetes. Each condition by itself increases the risk of developing serious health problems, such as cardiovascular disease, and so taking steps to address them is well worth the effort.

High blood pressure

Type 2 diabetes

Obesity

About **1 woman in 20** who becomes **pregnant** develops **gestational diabetes**

Secondary diabetes

Diabetes that results from another health problem or medical treatment is known as secondary diabetes. There are various possible causes, including viral infections that destroy insulin-producing cells in the pancreas; damage to the pancreas from conditions such as cystic fibrosis or pancreatitis; surgical removal of the pancreas; certain hormonal disorders, for example, Cushing's disease; or as a side effect of some medications, such as corticosteroids. The treatment varies according to the underlying cause.

Prediabetes

The term "prediabetes" refers to blood glucose that is slightly raised but not high enough to be classed as diabetes. If you are diagnosed with prediabetes, you can reduce your risk of developing type 2 diabetes with practical advice and support from your health professional (see pp.22–23).

Symptoms

The symptoms of type 1 and type 2 diabetes are similar, but they tend to come on suddenly in type 1 and develop gradually in type 2. To check whether your symptoms mean you have diabetes, it's important to have them checked by a doctor for a definite diagnosis (see pp.20–21).

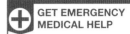

GET EMERGENCY MEDICAL HELP

If you or anyone else has intense thirst and any of the following:

- Nausea and vomiting; stomach pain; fruity-smelling breath; confusion; feeling faint or fainting; recent dramatic weight loss.

Recognizing diabetes

It is more common to be aware of the symptoms of high blood glucose if you have type 1 diabetes, because the absence of insulin has a dramatic effect on the body. If you have type 2 diabetes, you still produce some insulin, so your symptoms may be less severe – you may even attribute them to other causes, such as emotional stress or growing older. Some people who have type 2 diabetes do not have any noticeable symptoms and may not suspect that they have diabetes until it is detected in a routine medical or eye test, or a medical test for another health problem. Type 2 diabetes is also becoming more common in children and young people, so checking any symptoms with a health professional is important at any age.

You may feel **tired** all the time, **lose weight**, be constantly **thirsty**, and frequently pass large amounts of urine

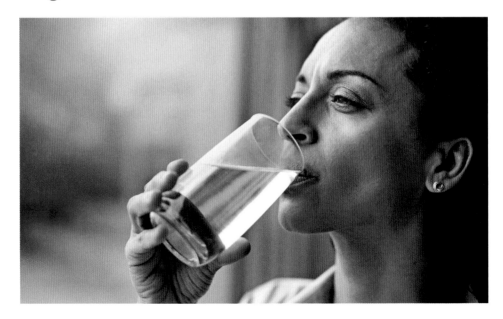

▷ **Constant thirst**
A common symptom of diabetes is feeling thirsty all the time, due to your kidneys producing large amounts of watery urine to filter out the excess glucose from your blood.

▽ **Possible symptoms of diabetes**

Diabetes can cause a wide range of symptoms, because it disrupts a vital aspect of body chemistry that affects all body cells. The main symptoms are similar in the most common types of diabetes – type 1 and type 2. The chief difference between the two is that symptoms tend to come on suddenly in type 1 but more gradually in type 2.

TIREDNESS AND LACK OF ENERGY

Because your cells are deprived of glucose – their main energy source – you may feel tired and lacking in energy all the time, even if you rest or sleep more than usual. You may also sometimes feel dizzy.

THIRST AND DRY MOUTH

Because you are passing a large amount of urine as part of your body's mechanism for reducing the level of glucose in your blood, you become dehydrated, which causes thirst and a dry mouth.

BLURRED VISION

When your blood glucose is raised, the lenses of your eyes absorb glucose and water. This makes them swell, causing blurred vision.

WEIGHT LOSS

When your body cannot use glucose, it starts to break down its fat and muscle stores for energy instead, so you may lose weight and muscle bulk. Weight loss is more common and rapid in type 1 diabetes. In type 2, weight loss may happen slowly or not at all.

PERSISTENT HUNGER

You may feel hungry much of the time, even shortly after eating, because the glucose from the digestion of food cannot enter your body cells due to the unavailability of insulin.

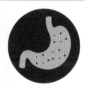

SLOW HEALING

Persistent raised blood glucose may lead to poor circulation of blood throughout the body. Because blood is needed to repair tissues, an impaired blood supply can slow down healing of damaged tissue, such as skin wounds.

FREQUENT, COPIOUS URINATION

When your blood glucose is too high, your kidneys filter out the excess glucose from your blood. To expel this excess glucose, your kidneys produce more urine.

SEXUAL DYSFUNCTION

Long-term raised blood glucose may lead to nerve damage and/or poor blood circulation. These, in turn, may cause problems such as erectile dysfunction in men or, in women, reduced sexual desire or painful intercourse.

CYSTITIS AND THRUSH

The glucose in your urine encourages bacteria and other microorganisms to grow in your urinary tract. This, in turn, may lead to infections such as cystitis (bladder infection) and thrush (infection of the vagina in women or penis in men), causing symptoms such as irritation around the penis or vagina.

Diagnosis

If you have symptoms that suggest you may have diabetes (see pp.18–19), you should consult your doctor because a definite diagnosis requires special tests to measure the level of glucose in your blood.

Types of tests

Initially, your doctor (or other health professional) may check a sample of your urine for glucose or give you a simple fingerprick blood test. These tests provide a result immediately. If glucose is detected in your urine or the fingerprick test indicates an unusually high blood glucose level, you will need one or more laboratory blood tests using a blood sample taken from a vein in your arm. Typically, these are a random blood glucose test, a fasting blood glucose test, and an oral glucose tolerance test.

In some instances, you may also be given a special test called a glycosylated haemoglobin test (HbA1c test, see p.31). This test provides a single measurement of your blood glucose that indicates what your average blood glucose level has been over the previous 2–3 months.

Blood glucose levels

The blood tests that are used to diagnose diabetes provide a measurement of the concentration of glucose in your blood – the amount of glucose in a specific volume of blood. The result – the blood glucose level – is given as millimoles of glucose per litre of blood; this is abbreviated as mmol/L. The blood tests also enable prediabetes (also called borderline diabetes) to be identified. In this condition, your blood glucose is slightly raised (6.1–6.9 mmol/L, as measured by a fasting blood glucose test) but is not high enough for diabetes to be diagnosed. However, a diagnosis of prediabetes indicates that you are at increased risk of developing type 2 diabetes, enabling you to take measures to help reduce your risk (see pp.22–23).

FASTING BLOOD GLUCOSE (NON-GESTATIONAL)

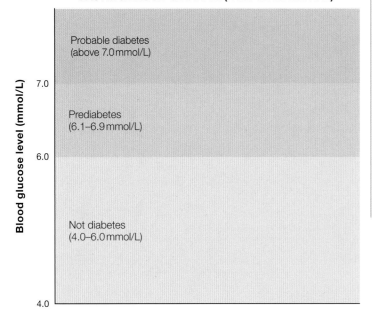

Blood glucose level (mmol/L)

Probable diabetes
(above 7.0 mmol/L)

7.0

Prediabetes
(6.1–6.9 mmol/L)

6.0

Not diabetes
(4.0–6.0 mmol/L)

4.0

◁ **Fasting blood glucose levels**
Your blood glucose level after fasting can indicate whether you do not have diabetes, or if you have prediabetes or diabetes.

MEDICAL TESTS USED IN THE DIAGNOSIS OF DIABETES

Although a urine or fingerprick test can reveal a raised blood glucose level, you need one or more of three laboratory blood tests to diagnose diabetes: the random or fasting blood glucose test and, if necessary, the oral glucose tolerance test. Your results are assessed with your symptoms. If you don't have any symptoms but diabetes is suspected, you need a repeat blood test carried out on a different day.

HOW THE TEST IS CARRIED OUT	WHAT THE RESULTS MEAN
Urine test A health professional tests a sample of your urine using a dipstick that changes colour according to the amount of glucose present. The dipstick is then compared to a colour chart to determine if glucose is present, and, if so, its level.	The presence or absence of glucose in the urine does not necessarily indicate or discount diabetes. If your urine contains glucose, or you have symptoms but no glucose, you will be referred for further blood tests.
Fingerprick test A health professional uses a device to prick the side of your fingertip and obtain a drop of blood. The blood drop is put onto a testing strip already inserted in a blood glucose meter, which provides a reading of your blood glucose level.	A healthy blood glucose level is in the range of 4–6 mmol/L. If your test result is above 6 mmol/L, your health professional will ask you to have further blood tests. A fingerprick test by itself is not enough to diagnose diabetes.
Random blood glucose test Your health professional takes a blood sample from your arm to send to a laboratory for analysis. This sample can be taken regardless of whether or not you have eaten.	If you have symptoms and your blood glucose result is above 11.1 mmol/L, you are diagnosed with diabetes. If you have no symptoms, or the result is lower than this, you may have a repeat test while fasting or be given an oral glucose tolerance test.
Fasting blood glucose test You do not eat or drink (except water) overnight, and in the morning your health professional takes a blood sample from your arm. The sample is sent to a laboratory for analysis.	If you have symptoms and your blood glucose result is above 7 mmol/L, you are diagnosed with diabetes; for a diagnosis of gestational diabetes, your blood glucose level must be above 5.6 mmol/L. If you have no symptoms, or the result is lower and you have symptoms, you may have a repeat test or be given an oral glucose tolerance test.
Oral glucose tolerance test You do not eat or drink (except water) overnight and in the morning your health professional takes a blood sample from your arm. You are then given a glucose drink, and 2 hours later your health professional takes another blood sample from your arm. The samples are sent for analysis.	If your fasting blood glucose level is 7 mmol/L or higher and/or your 2-hour test result is above 11.1 mmol/L, you are diagnosed with diabetes, whether or not you have symptoms; for a diagnosis of gestational diabetes, the 2-hour level must be 7.8 mmol/L or higher. This test is used when other tests have been inconclusive or if you have risk factors for diabetes.

Preventing and reversing diabetes

For many people with type 2 diabetes, reversal (also called remission or suppression) of their diabetes is possible through weight loss and increased activity. These measures can also often help to prevent prediabetes from progressing to type 2 diabetes. Other types of diabetes cannot yet be prevented or reversed, although careful diabetes management can help to minimize their effects.

Prediabetes and type 2 diabetes

In prediabetes, also called borderline diabetes, your blood glucose is raised but not high enough to be classed as diabetes. It is an indication that you are at high risk of developing type 2 diabetes.

If you have prediabetes, it is possible to prevent or delay the onset of type 2 diabetes by losing weight, if you weigh more than the recommended healthy weight for your height (see pp.92–93), and becoming more active. The same measures may also help to reverse type 2 diabetes in the early years after

diagnosis or, at any time, reduce or delay the need for medication. If you do not have prediabetes or type 2 diabetes but are concerned that you may develop them, you can reduce your risk by maintaining a healthy weight, following healthy eating principles, and being physically active on a regular basis.

Other types of diabetes

Type 1 diabetes, MODY (maturity onset diabetes of the young), and LADA (latent autoimmune diabetes in adults) cannot yet be cured, prevented, or reversed. However, maintaining a healthy weight, eating healthily, and being physically active can help to manage the conditions and prevent complications.

CHILDREN AND YOUNG PEOPLE

Type 1 diabetes Research is being carried out into ways of delaying the onset of type 1 diabetes in younger groups at risk of developing it, but the research is still at an early stage of development.

Type 2 diabetes Methods for preventing this type of diabetes, minimizing its effects, or putting it into remission for children and young people are the same as those for adults: weight loss and increased activity. Specialist help from health professionals is vital, together with emotional and practical support for the whole family.

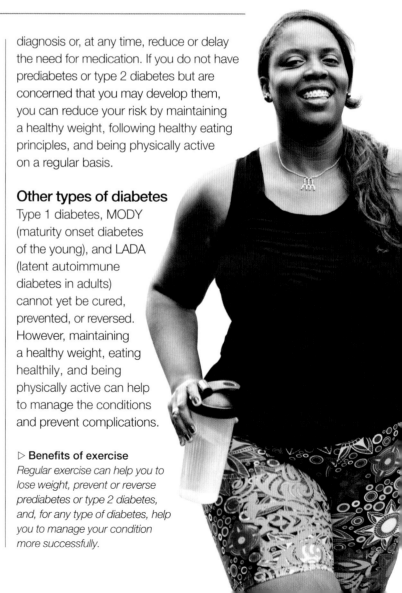

▷ **Benefits of exercise**
Regular exercise can help you to lose weight, prevent or reverse prediabetes or type 2 diabetes, and, for any type of diabetes, help you to manage your condition more successfully.

If you develop gestational diabetes, it may disappear after you have given birth, although it indicates that you are at high risk of developing type 2 diabetes. You can help to minimize this risk by maintaining a healthy weight and eating pattern.

Practical measures

For information on measures to lose weight (if necessary), see pp.94–99, and for suggestions about becoming more active, see pp.100–103. Together, weight loss and increased physical activity reduce the amount of internal fat around your liver and pancreas, which increases the efficiency of insulin production. Reducing internal fat also counteracts insulin resistance by increasing your body cells' response to insulin. In addition, these measures help to reduce health risks associated with diabetes, such as heart disease, and physical actvity can help to reduce stress and boost your mood.

Preventing or reversing type 2 diabetes means that you have reduced your blood glucose level into the non-diabetes range. However, this does not mean that you have been cured. There is the risk that your prediabetes or type 2 diabetes will return – for example, if you regain lost weight – and for this reason, you will still need regular health reviews.

Losing weight and becoming more active can be very challenging. You will be more successful if you have clear, realistic goals, an action plan, and encouragement. Ask your health professional for personalized support to help you achieve your goals. If you have

The **keys** to **prevention** or **reversal** are **losing weight** and becoming **more active**

prediabetes or type 2 diabetes, you may also be offered a programme* to help you prevent or reverse your diabetes.

Weight-loss surgery

Also called bariatric surgery, weight-loss surgery is not usually recommended for diabetes unless you have type 2 diabetes, are very overweight, and have been unable to lose weight by any other means. There are various procedures, but they all either reduce the size of your stomach or re-route part of your digestive tract to bypass the stomach and/or part of the intestine. The most common method is gastric banding, which is reversible, unlike other types of bariatric surgery. Surgery can be effective in reversing type 2 diabetes, reducing blood pressure and blood lipid levels (such as blood cholesterol levels), and improving your health and quality of life in the long term. However, weight-loss surgery is not suitable for everybody and, like all surgery, carries the risk of complications and adverse effects.

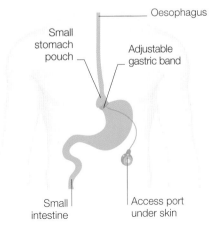

Oesophagus

Small stomach pouch

Adjustable gastric band

Small intestine

Access port under skin

◁ **Gastric banding**
In this type of bariatric surgery, the size of the stomach is reduced by placing an inflatable band around the upper part of the stomach. The band can be tightened by injecting liquid into it through an access port implanted just under the skin.

What to expect when first diagnosed

A diagnosis of diabetes can affect your life in many ways. It may affect you emotionally and will also have practical effects on your everyday life as you learn to manage your condition. You will have various medical checks, meet a range of health professionals, and receive a great deal of advice and information about adjusting to life with diabetes.

Medical checks and treatment

If initial checks or symptoms indicate that you may have diabetes, the diagnosis will need to be confirmed using special tests (see pp.20–21) by a doctor. If the diagnosis is confirmed, you will have additional medical checks to assess other aspects of your health, such as your eye health, heart and circulation, and nerve function. These checks also provide a baseline for your future annual reviews, which will include the same checks (see pp.142–143). The initial checks are also useful for detecting any health issues that need immediate treatment or monitoring.

Along with the medical checks, you will be prescribed initial treatment for your diabetes, either insulin or other medication. If you have type 1 diabetes, you will be referred urgently to a specialist clinic, where you will learn how to manage insulin; for the first few weeks, you will also have frequent – possibly daily – contact with the clinic staff. If you have type 2 diabetes, you will continue to attend your GP's clinic regularly to establish the type and amount of diabetes medication you need and monitor your progress. If necessary, you may also be prescribed other medication, for example, to reduce raised blood pressure.

Your initial care will also include a consultation with a dietitian about your food in relation to your diabetes, and with other health professionals to provide any immediate practical advice you may need, such as help with blood glucose monitoring.

MEDICAL CHECKS ON DIAGNOSIS

Height and weight measurement to calculate your body mass index (see p.93).

Blood pressure measurement and checking your heart health with a stethoscope

Examination of your legs and feet to check your blood circulation and sensation

Retinal photography to check the health of your retina (the light-sensitive layer in your eyes)

Blood tests to check your glucose levels (with the HbA1c test, see p.31); blood lipids, such as cholesterol; thyroid function; liver function; and kidney function

Coming to terms with living with diabetes means exploring your feelings as much as taking insulin or other medication

Working with health professionals

Diabetes care is optimal when you and your health professionals work together as a team, with you as the expert on your own life and health and them as experts on the medical aspects of the condition. This approach is known as individualized care planning, and it begins right from diagnosis.

When you are first diagnosed, you will be offered a diabetes education course to learn more about the condition, ask questions, and meet others who are also newly diagnosed. The courses are run by diabetes health professionals. The timing and length of the courses vary, but the content is similar and includes information about diabetes itself, food, treatments, and how to keep healthy. For people who have type 1 diabetes, carbohydrate counting (see p.82), adjusting insulin doses (see pp.48–51), and dealing with hypoglycaemia (see pp.62–67) are also covered. If you have any concerns about attending a course, your health professional can provide your education personally or make arrangements that are convenient for you.

Emotional support

When you are first diagnosed with diabetes, it can take time to adjust emotionally. You will be asked about your feelings during your early consultations and given the chance to talk about them. This is important because your feelings can influence how well you are able to manage your diabetes so that you stay healthy (see pp.110–111). You may also find it helpful to join a diabetes support group, whether you have diabetes yourself or are responsible for someone who has diabetes. When you are first diagnosed, trying out a local or online support group – peer support – will help you work out whether the group is useful for you. Your health professional can also give you information about support groups.

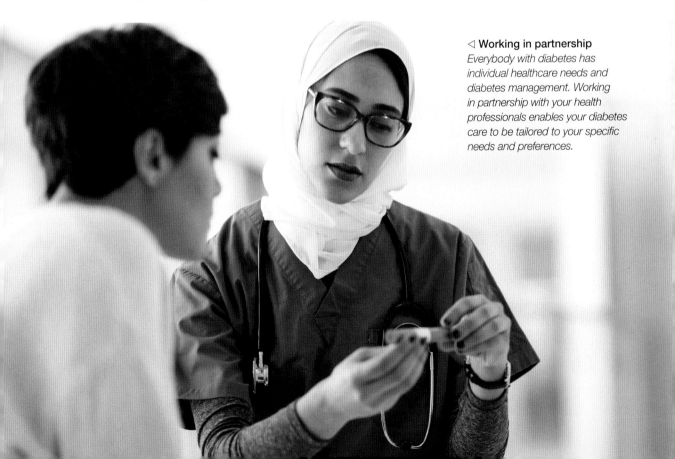

◁ **Working in partnership**
Everybody with diabetes has individual healthcare needs and diabetes management. Working in partnership with your health professionals enables your diabetes care to be tailored to your specific needs and preferences.

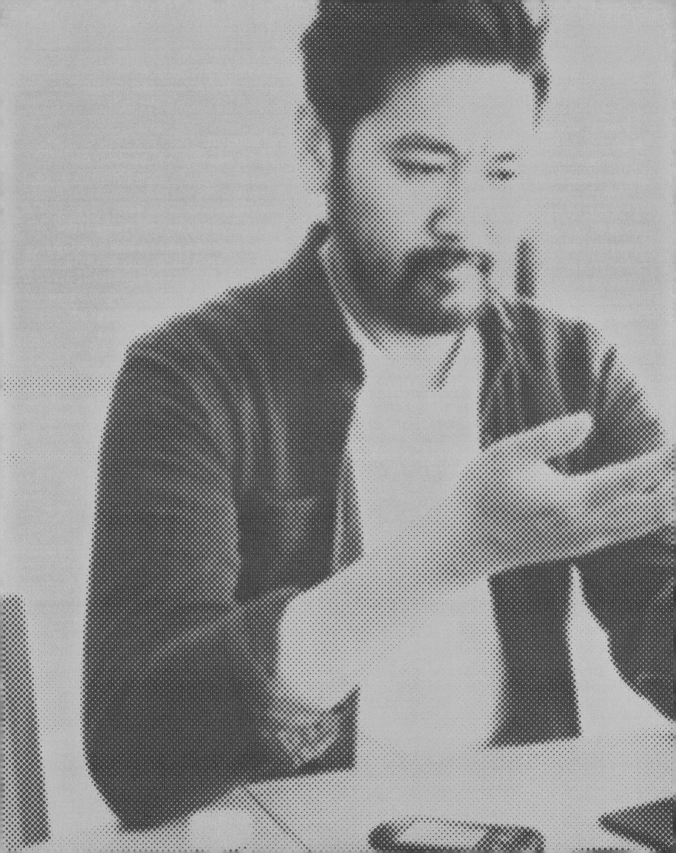

Managing your blood glucose

Monitoring blood glucose

Regularly monitoring the amount of glucose in your blood is a key part of the daily care of your diabetes. The results give you information about how your blood glucose is responding to treatment, so you can adjust it if necessary. To manage your blood glucose effectively, it can help if you understand what level you are aiming for and factors that can affect it.

Understanding blood glucose levels

Your blood glucose level is a figure that indicates the concentration of glucose in your blood. The level is given as millimoles of glucose per litre of blood (abbreviated to mmol/L). Your blood glucose level naturally changes throughout the day. For people without diabetes, their body keeps the level within a constant range, usually 4–7 mmol/L. For people with diabetes, their body cannot maintain the glucose level effectively and the changes tend to be larger and more frequent.

Types and aims of monitoring

There are two main types of monitoring: self checks of your blood glucose level, which you do every day, and measuring your HbA1c (glycosylated haemoglobin) level, which is carried out by your healthcare professional at regular intervals.

The aim of self checks is to give you information about the effects of the factors that can affect your blood glucose level, such a food, drink, activity, and medication. If you change your diabetes treatment, monitoring your blood glucose will give you vital feedback on how well the treatment is working. Self-checks can also tell you if your blood glucose is low (hypoglycaemia, see pp.62–67) or raised (hyperglycaemia, see pp.68–71), and can help you to manage special situations, such as illness. The HbA1c test gives a measure of your blood glucose level over the previous 2 or 3 months.

> **If you change your diabetes treatment, monitoring your blood glucose will give you vital feedback on how well the treatment is working**

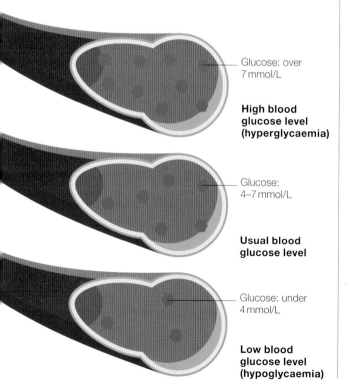

Glucose: over
7 mmol/L

**High blood
glucose level
(hyperglycaemia)**

Glucose:
4–7 mmol/L

**Usual blood
glucose level**

Glucose: under
4 mmol/L

**Low blood
glucose level
(hypoglycaemia)**

▷ **Blood glucose checking**
Using a lancet to obtain a drop of blood from your finger for checking your blood glucose level with a meter is simple to do and can usually be fitted into your everyday activities. This fingerprick method provides an accurate snapshot of your blood glucose level at that time.

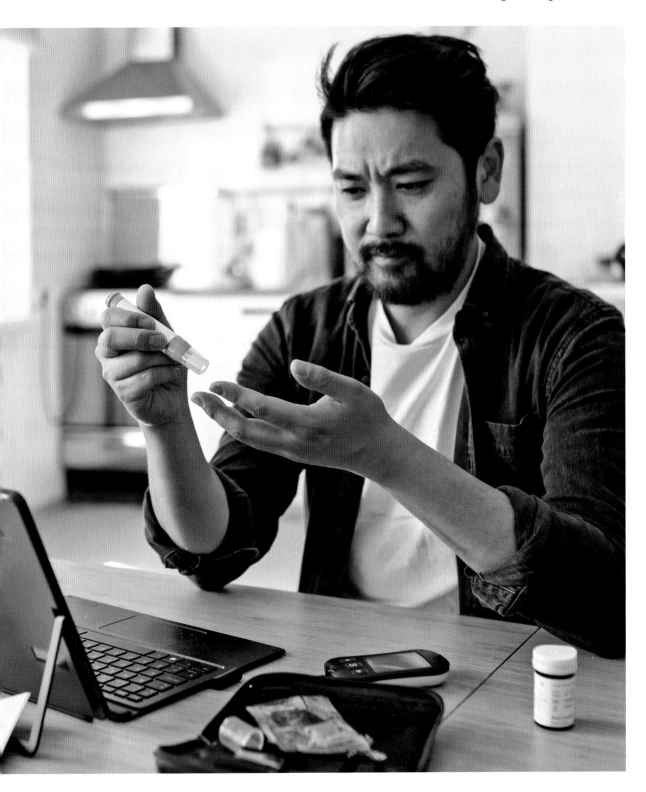

Recommended blood glucose levels

Whatever type of diabetes you have, as a general rule of thumb, it is recommended that you aim to keep your blood glucose within the range 4–9 mmol/L. This is close to the blood glucose range of a person without diabetes (4–7 mmol/L). A blood glucose level that is in the recommended range will keep you feeling well and help to prevent possible long-term complications. Although a blood glucose level of 4–9 mmol/L is a general recommendation, you and your healthcare professional may agree on different target ranges that are appropriate for you personally. In addition, you may be given different recommended targets in specific circumstances; for example, if you have difficulty recognizing a hypo or if you are planning a pregnancy.

Frequency of checks

If you have type 1 diabetes, you will be advised to check your blood glucose between 4 and 10 times a day. If you have type 2 diabetes, you may not need to check your own blood glucose levels, except if you are taking medication that includes an insulin-stimulating drug, such as a sulphonylurea (see pp.58–59)

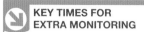

KEY TIMES FOR EXTRA MONITORING

Monitoring your blood glucose is always important, but there are certain times when you need to check more often.

- During and for several hours after vigorous or long periods of exercise.
- If you have an unpredictable working pattern or do shift work.
- If you change your medication and/or insulin regimen.
- When planning a pregnancy and during the pregnancy itself.
- When you are ill.
- If you have been drinking alcohol or using recreational drugs.
- During holidays and celebrations.

and/or insulin (see pp.42–43), because of the risk of hypoglycaemia with these treatments. In this case, typically you will be advised to check your blood glucose routinely twice a day.

Whatever type of diabetes you have, if you are particularly concerned about hypos while you are sleeping, you may be advised to check your blood glucose level during the night. There are other times and situations in which your blood glucose level is likely to vary or you are at particular risk of a hypo and you will need to do extra checks (see box, above).

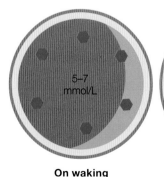

5–7 mmol/L

On waking

4–7 mmol/L

Before meals

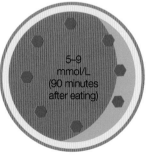

5–9 mmol/L (90 minutes after eating)

After meals

◁ **Typical recommended targets**
Blood glucose levels to aim for vary according to your age, the type of diabetes you have and the time of day. The examples given here are of typical targets for an adult with type 1 diabetes but your personal targets may be different.

If you normally check your blood glucose level, you will also need to make sure you check it before you drive and at frequent intervals while you are driving (see pp.114–115).

Self-monitoring

There are various methods of checking your own blood glucose levels. The simplest is a urine test, in which a glucose-sensitive test strip is dipped in a sample of urine. The strip changes colour according to the concentration of glucose in the urine, and the colour of the strip is compared against a chart to give a reading of the blood glucose level. This method may be used by healthcare professionals but home urine testing is not very accurate and is not generally recommended.

The most common method for self-checking is with the fingerprick method, in which a drop of blood is obtained by pricking your finger with a lancet, then applying the blood to a strip that is analysed by a blood glucose meter to give a reading of your blood glucose level (see pp.36–37). Other methods include using a continuous blood glucose monitor, which provides continuous readings of you glucose level using a sensor under the skin (see pp.35 and 37), and flash monitoring, which provides readings using a skin sensor and separate scanner (see pp.35 and 37).

The HbA1c test

Also sometimes called the glycosylated haemoglobin test, this test relies on the fact that, in the blood, glucose joins to haemoglobin (the oxygen-carrying component of blood), forming a substance known as glycosylated haemoglobin, or HbA1c. The level of HbA1c is not significantly affected by recent food intake,

▷ **Glycosylated haemoglobin**
In red blood cells, glucose joins to haemoglobin to form glycosylated haemoglobin, or HbA1c. The level of HbA1c indicates longer-term blood glucose levels.

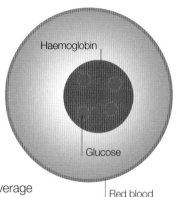

Haemoglobin

Glucose

Red blood cell

so it provides a picture of your average blood glucose level over the previous 2 or 3 months and gives an indication of how well your diabetes treatment is working. The test usually involves laboratory analysis of a blood sample taken from a vein in your arm or by a portable fingerprick meter. Typically, you will be offered an HbA1c check by a health professional every 3 to 6 months, whether or not you self-monitor your blood glucose levels.

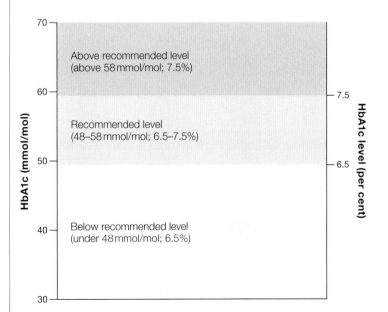

△ **Recommended HbA1c level**
The recommended level of HbA1c is 48–58 mmol/mol (also sometimes given as 6.5–7.5%), although you and your health professional may agree a personal target range.

Monitoring equipment

Special equipment is available to enable you to check your blood glucose level. The most common method is fingerprick checking. This involves using a lancing device and lancet to obtain a drop of blood, which is then put on a test strip that has been inserted in a blood glucose meter. Other methods are continuous glucose monitoring and flash monitoring, which utilize sensors in the skin.

Lancing devices and lancets

A lancing device is a hand-held device containing a spring and a lancet. Each lancet consists of a plastic body containing a needle, which has has a protective cap over its end. Each lancet is designed to be used only once. There are different designs of lancing devices but they all typically have the same basic features: a control that enables you to alter the depth to which the lancet penetrates your skin; a priming button that compresses the spring ready for firing the lancet's needle; and a release button that fires the needle.

To obtain a drop of blood for a glucose check, you remove the protective end cap from the lancing device, insert a lancet, and adjust the depth dial to alter how deep the lancet needle penetrates (see illustration opposite). Then you prime the device, hold it against your finger, and press the release button to fire the lancet. Once you have completed your blood glucose check, you remove and dispose of the lancet in a medical sharps box. With single-use lancing devices, typically you only need to remove the cover, place the device against your finger, then press the release mechanism.

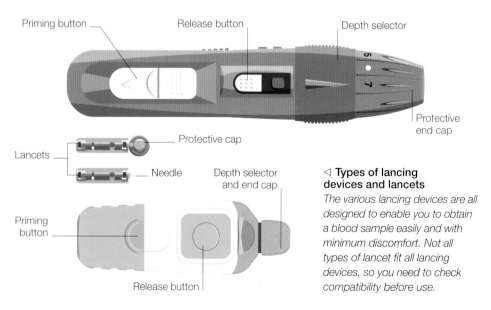

Priming button — Release button — Depth selector

Lancets — Protective cap — Needle

Priming button — Depth selector and end cap — Release button

Protective end cap

◁ **Types of lancing devices and lancets**
The various lancing devices are all designed to enable you to obtain a blood sample easily and with minimum discomfort. Not all types of lancet fit all lancing devices, so you need to check compatibility before use.

INSTALLING A FRESH LANCET

Different lancing devices vary in their design, features, and precise method of installing a fresh lancet. The general method shown here is applicable to many types of lancet, but you should refer to the manufacturer's instructions for specific information about installing a lancet for your particular device.

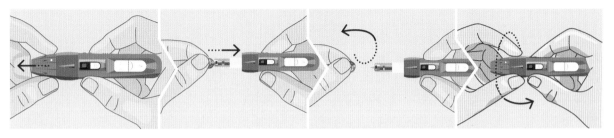

1 Remove the end cap from the lancing device. This will expose the socket into which you will insert a fresh lancet.

2 Take a fesh lancet and insert it into the exposed socket of the lancing device. Make sure you push the lancet in as far as it will go.

3 Twist off the lancet's protective cap to expose the needle. Take care not to contaminate the needle by allowing it to touch anything.

4 Carefully replace the end cap of the lancing device and twist the depth selector to adjust how deep the needle will penetrate.

Test strips

A glucose test strip is inserted into a blood glucose meter and then a drop of blood is applied to the end of the strip. A chemical in the strip reacts with glucose to produce a small electric current, which is detected by the meter and converted into a reading of your blood glucose level. Test strips are available in pots of 25 or 50 strips, or individually packed. The strip you use must be new and within its expiry date. If you use a strip from a pot, replace the top immediately to protect the remaining strips.

▽ **Blood glucose test strips**
Test strips are small, disposable pieces of plastic containing a chemical that reacts with glucose in blood. Most strips are designed to be used by one type of meter.

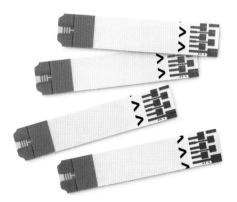

SAFE DISPOSAL OF USED EQUIPMENT

It is important that your used lancets and test strips are disposed of safely. They should be put in a medical sharps box. A sharps box should also be used for disposable needles and syringes. Once an item has been put in the box, do not try to take it out again. The box should be kept in a safe place, out of the sight and reach of children. When full, the box should be sealed and disposed of according to the arrangements for your particular area. Your health professionals will be able to advise you about these.

Blood glucose meters

These are small, battery-operated devices that measure and display the level of glucose in a small sample of blood on the test strip (see Checking your blood glucose, pp.36–37). The display appears in a few seconds. You can then record the result, add it to the meter memory, or download it. There are many different meters available, with a range of functions and features. You will be given one by your health professional if they advise you to check your blood glucose level, or you can choose to buy one, or a spare one.

From time to time, it is advisable to check the accuracy of your meter. This simply involves using a control solution with a known level of glucose instead of a blood sample.

CHOOSING THE RIGHT METER

There are a number of aspects to consider when you are working out which is the right meter for you. As well as the points listed below, you might also want to consider the cost and/or availability of the test strips a particular meter uses.

SIZE	A compact meter is more convenient to carry, but if you have a condition that affects your dexterity, such as arthritis, you may find a larger meter easier to use.
SIZE OF BLOOD SAMPLE	The amount of blood you need to put on a test strip to obtain an accurate reading can vary according to the equipment you use. If you find it difficult to obtain blood, it may help to choose a meter that needs only a small sample.
DISPLAY	A meter with a large display may be easier to read. Some meters show the reading on its own, others display additonal information as well. More sophisticated meters enable you to customize the display.
MEMORY	Meters vary in the number of readings they can store. A large memory is useful if you cannot record or download the readings.
DOWNLOADING	Some meters allow you to download your readings and analyse them on a computer or smartphone. This enables you to see your blood glucose levels over a period in graph or table form.
AVERAGES	Many meters can give you an average of your readings over the past week or longer.
TIMING	Meters vary in how quickly they display readings. A meter with a shorter analysis time may make it easier for you to do a blood glucose check when you are busy.
ADVANCED FEATURES	Some meters can measure both blood glucose and blood ketones. Others can hold multiple test strips so you do not need to insert one every time you use it. Some high-tech meters contain built-in software that provides various analysis and/or display options.

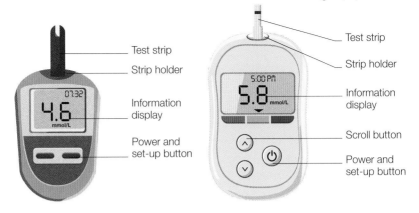

▷ **Varieties of meters**

Blood glucose meters are available in various sizes and shapes and with different added features to suit individual requirements. They all have to meet minimum standards for accuracy. Like all electronic devices, they should be kept clean and dry. Most types use standard batteries, although some models are rechargeable.

Test strip
Strip holder
Information display
Power and set-up button

Test strip
Strip holder
Information display
Scroll button
Power and set-up button

Continuous glucose monitors

A CGM consists of a sensor, transmitter, and receiver (a hand-held reader or a combined reader and insulin pump). The sensor, which is fitted into the skin, measures glucose in the fluid around the cells below your skin (known as interstitial fluid). The glucose level in this fluid mirrors the level in your blood but there might be a short time lag before the CGM reading accurately reflects your blood glucose level.

Flash monitors

Similar to a continuous glucose monitor, a flash monitor consists of a sensor fitted into the skin and a separate scanner that displays your blood glucose reading. As with a CGM, the sensor of a flash monitor measures the glucose level in interstitial fluid, which is then converted into a reading of your blood glucose level. Instead of a scanner, you can also use a compatible smartphone that has the correct app.

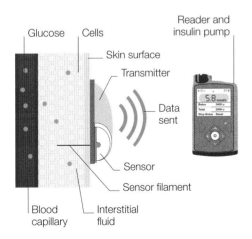

Glucose
Cells
Reader and insulin pump
Skin surface
Transmitter
Data sent
Sensor
Sensor filament
Blood capillary
Interstitial fluid

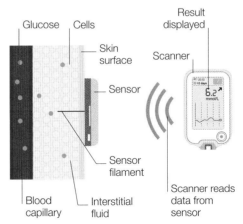

Glucose
Cells
Result displayed
Skin surface
Scanner
Sensor
Sensor filament
Scanner reads data from sensor
Blood capillary
Interstitial fluid

△ **How a continuous glucose monitor works**
A sensor detects glucose in interstitial fluid. A transmitter automatically sends data about the glucose level to a reader, which displays your blood glucose level, or to a combined reader and pump, which can also manage your insulin dose.

△ **How a flash monitor works**
A flash monitor works in a similar way to a continuous glucose monitor. However, a flash monitor does not have a transmitter. You need to scan the sensor to obtain a reading of your blood glucose level.

Checking your blood glucose

There are various ways of checking your blood glucose. The commonly used fingerprick method gives an accurate "snapshot" reading of your glucose level. Other checking options are to use a flash monitor or a continuous glucose monitor.

Fingerprick method

This procedure gives you an immediate reading of your blood glucose level. For fingerprick readings, you need three items of equipment. The first is a lancing device for pricking your finger to get a drop of blood. This device fires a small needle, known as a lancet, into your skin; you can set the depth to which the lancet will pierce your skin. The second item is a blood glucose meter. The third is a set of test strips. You insert one end of a strip into the meter and collect a drop of your blood on the other end. The meter analyses the information from the blood on the strip to produce a reading of your blood glucose level. You also need a sharps bin to dispose of used lancets.

DOING A FINGERPRICK CHECK

The usual site for taking a blood sample is the side of your fingertip, not too close to the nail. (Less commonly, you may need to take blood from your forearm, the palm of your hand, or your abdomen, if your equipment is designed to take blood from these sites.) Take care to follow the manufacturer's instructions on how to use your meter correctly. It may help to rub your hand from the palm towards your fingers to get the blood flowing.

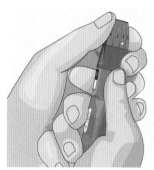 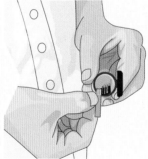 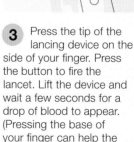 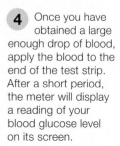

1 Wash and dry your hands. With a fresh lancet in your lancing device, turn the device's dial to your preferred depth level. Low numbers indicate a shallow depth; higher numbers mean that the lancet will penetrate deeper.

2 Take a fresh test strip from its container. Switch on your blood glucose meter or insert the test strip into the meter to switch it on, depending on the manufacturer's instructions for your specific meter.

3 Press the tip of the lancing device on the side of your finger. Press the button to fire the lancet. Lift the device and wait a few seconds for a drop of blood to appear. (Pressing the base of your finger can help the blood flow.)

4 Once you have obtained a large enough drop of blood, apply the blood to the end of the test strip. After a short period, the meter will display a reading of your blood glucose level on its screen.

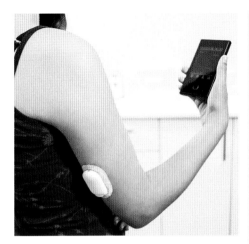

△ **Using a continuous glucose monitor**
Attach the sensor and transmitter to your skin.
These continually send blood glucose data to a
separate monitor, which displays your readings.

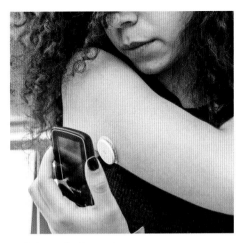

△ **Using a flash monitor**
To obtain a reading, hold your flash reader or
smartphone (if it has the correct app) over the
sensor. The data will appear on the screen.

Continuous glucose monitoring

A CGM measures your glucose level continually, and you can choose to see your readings immediately (real-time CGM) or can download a set of readings every day (retrospective CGM). A CGM can also be set up to alert you if your blood glucose becomes too high or low. Because a CGM measures glucose in the interstitial fluid (see p.35), you still need to do a fingerprick check if you need immediate information about your blood glucose level. You will also need to do one or two fingerprick checks a day to ensure the CGM readings remain accurate. Some CGMs can also link to an insulin pump, to manage your insulin dose (see pp.54–55).

Flash monitoring

Like a CGM, a flash monitor measures your blood glucose continually. However, unlike with a CGM, you have to manually scan the sensor to see your readings. As well as your blood glucose level, the display also has an arrow to indicate whether your blood glucose level is stable, rising, or falling. Flash monitors also have a memory feature, but they do not have an alarm that will alert you if your blood glucose level falls outside your recommended range. It is also not possible to link them to an insulin pump. As with CGMs, you will need to do a fingerprick check from time to time to check the accuracy of readings.

RECORDING LEVELS

It is useful to keep a record of your glucose readings so that you can see changes over time. You can record the figures in a written diary, but many blood glucose monitoring systems enble you to upload results for storage and analysis on a smartphone, tablet, or computer. Also keep notes about your food, medication doses, and activities so that you can relate these to your blood glucose readings.

What your results may mean

Examining your blood glucose results over a period of days or weeks can give you vital information about how well you are managing your blood glucose level and what action, if any, you need to take in response.

Responding to results

It is better to look for patterns in your blood glucose readings than to focus on the occasional high or low reading. If you can view the figures as a graph or table, it is easier to spot trends: for example, whether your reading tends to be high or low at a particular time of day. The ideal range for your blood glucose is 4–9 millimoles per litre (mmol/L). If your results are rarely or never in this range or constantly fluctuate, try taking corrective action, such as changing your food, activity level, or medication dose. If these measures don't work, speak to your health professional as you may need a change in your medication and/or insulin regimen.

▷ **Checking results**
Some monitors can display results as a graph or chart, or can upload them to a computer or mobile device, such as a smartphone, to enable you to see the results graphically and spot trends in your glucose readings.

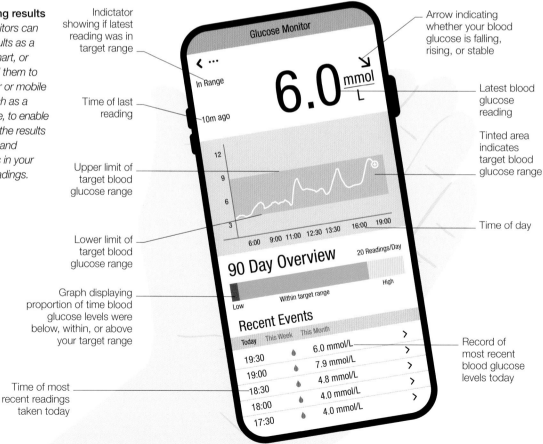

Indictator showing if latest reading was in target range

Arrow indicating whether your blood glucose is falling, rising, or stable

Time of last reading

Latest blood glucose reading

Tinted area indicates target blood glucose range

Upper limit of target blood glucose range

Lower limit of target blood glucose range

Time of day

Graph displaying proportion of time blood glucose levels were below, within, or above your target range

Time of most recent readings taken today

Record of most recent blood glucose levels today

Glucose Monitor

In Range

10m ago

6.0 mmol/L

12
9
6
3

6:00 9:00 11:00 12:30 13:30 16:00 19:00

90 Day Overview   20 Readings/Day

Low   Within target range   High

Recent Events

Today   This Week   This Month

19:30   6.0 mmol/L
19:00   7.9 mmol/L
18:30   4.8 mmol/L
18:00   4.0 mmol/L
17:30   4.0 mmol/L

Higher blood glucose readings

In practice, a single raised reading with no obvious cause happens from time to time and does not need any action. However, if your readings are constantly raised over a day or more, you need to find the cause and take appropriate action. For example, if stress or illness raises your blood glucose for more than one or two days, you can temporarily increase your medication. If you have put on weight, you may need to increase your medication to counteract the insulin resistance this causes. Subsequent blood glucose levels will show how successful your actions have been. (For more about hyperglycaemia, see pp.68–69.)

Lower blood glucose readings

Blood glucose levels below 4 mmol/L indicate hypoglycaemia and need to be treated immediately (see pp.66–67). If your levels often fall below 4 mmol/L, this can reduce your awareness of the signs of a hypo. If you have had a hypo, work out the cause and then closely monitor your blood glucose levels to enable you to plan ahead to help maintain your target blood glucose levels.

Rather than focusing on the occasional high or low result, look for patterns

COMMON CAUSES OF HIGHS AND LOWS

An occasional out-of-range blood glucose level does not indicate that you need to make changes (although a low blood glucose level should always be treated promptly). However, if you notice a pattern of highs or lows, or constant fluctuations, finding out why can help you take corrective action.

HIGHER READINGS	LOWER READINGS
Having more food than usual or a different type of food. (A specific food may be a cause if it's associated with high readings on several occasions.)	Having less food than usual, or taking your insulin and/or medication and then being unable to eat at the planned time.
Being less physically active than usual.	Being more physically active than usual.
Illness can cause a high blood glucose reading, as can stress hormones.	Stress can make your blood glucose level fall if you respond to it by using up more energy or eating less than usual.
Forgetting to take your medication or your insulin or taking an insufficient dose.	Taking an extra dose of medication, injecting more than your usual dose of insulin, or being on too high a dose of medication or insulin.
Putting on weight.	Losing weight.
Special circumstances, such as having a hypo earlier in the day, which you treated with glucose (when you are hypo, your liver also converts glycogen into glucose and releases the glucose into your bloodstream).	Special circumstances, such as drinking a lot of alcohol without compensating by eating carbohydrate-containing food at the same time or reducing your dosage of medication.

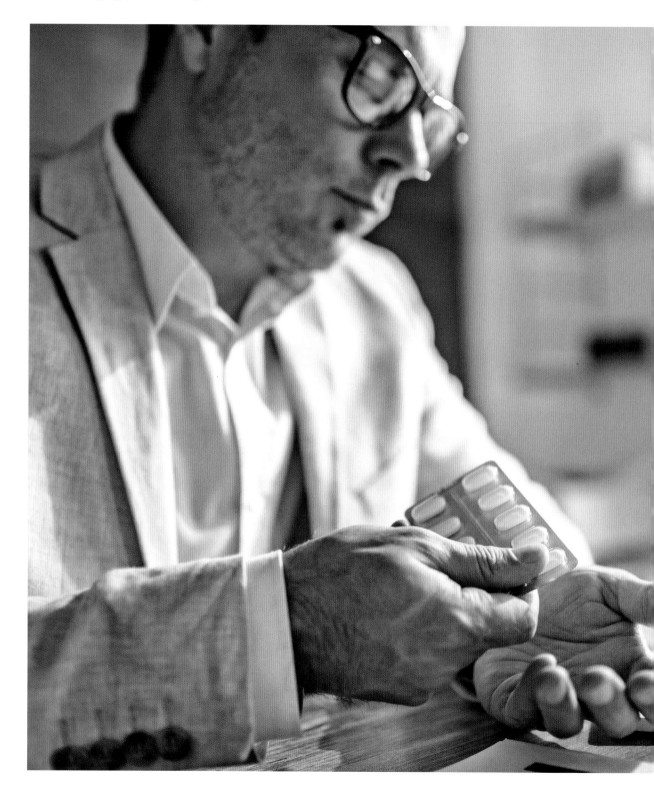

◁ **Diabetes tablets**
The many types of tablets for type 2 diabetes help in day-to-day management of blood glucose levels.

Medication for diabetes

Medication will help you to manage your blood glucose levels, but which treatment will depend on the type of diabetes, along with other factors. If you have type 1 diabetes, you will need insulin; type 2 diabetes is usually treated with tablets and lifestyle changes, if you need them. Insulin or non-insulin injectable drugs can be added too.

Who needs medication?

Anyone diagnosed as having type 1 diabetes will have to start taking insulin straight away. If you are diagnosed with type 2 diabetes, you are likely to start on tablets, although you may eventually need insulin too if tablets alone don't keep your blood glucose levels within a healthy range. The point at which treatment starts for type 2 diabetes depends on whether you have symptoms and on your blood glucose level.

Good management of your diabetes with insulin or tablets will help to slow or halt the development of complications, for example, eye and kidney problems (see pp.176–201).

Insulin treatment

Insulin is always taken by injection or delivered via a pump (see pp.52–55) so that it can get straight into your bloodstream. Insulin can't be taken as a tablet because it would be destroyed by your digestive system. Most of the insulin used today is human or analogue insulin, which means it has been manufactured in a laboratory to work in a way similar to the insulin produced by a human pancreas. If you have had diabetes for many years, you may still be taking animal insulin (usually derived from pig pancreas). However, this is less commonly used and is no longer likely to be prescribed as a first choice of insulin. See pp.42–57 for more information about insulin treatment.

Tablets and other medication

Used to help manage type 2 diabetes, tablets work mainly by enabling body cells to take up and use naturally produced insulin effectively or by stimulating the pancreas to produce more insulin. If you have type 2 diabetes, your health professional will assess which tablet may suit you best and discuss the choices with you.

Incretin mimetics (GLP-1 receptor agonists), like insulin, have to be taken as an injection. These drugs increase insulin release from the pancreas in response to food and also make you feel fuller earlier into a meal, thus helping you to control how much you eat.

People with type 2 diabetes may need both tablets and insulin to manage their diabetes and keep healthy

Insulin treatment

Insulin is essential when you have type 1 diabetes and is likely to be part of your treatment at some point when you have type 2 diabetes. There are many types and regimens of insulin (see pp.44–47), and these can be adapted and the doses adjusted to help you get the best fit for your diabetes and your day-to-day life.

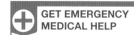

GET EMERGENCY MEDICAL HELP

- Taking too much insulin can lead to hypoglycaemia (see pp.62–67). This may be severe, especially if you haven't eaten recently or are drinking alcohol. In these circumstances, getting emergency help is essential.

Who needs insulin?

Insulin is an essential hormone – without it your body cells cannot take in glucose from your blood to use for energy. If your pancreas no longer produces insulin, or it produces so little that the medication you take for diabetes is no longer effective, you will need an external source of insulin, usually in the form of regular injections prescribed by your health professional.

If you have type 1 diabetes, your life depends on receiving insulin by injection or insulin pump. If you have type 2 diabetes or MODY (see p.17), and your blood glucose level consistently rises above the recommended ranges with other types of medication, you will also be prescribed insulin.

Insulin may also be needed on a short-term basis – for example, if you go into hospital for a major operation and can't eat and drink. Women who have type 2 diabetes will sometimes need to switch from tablets to insulin if they become pregnant. Some women with gestational diabetes (see pp.136–137) need insulin while pregnant if changes to food intake and activity level do not keep blood glucose levels within the ideal range for pregnancy.

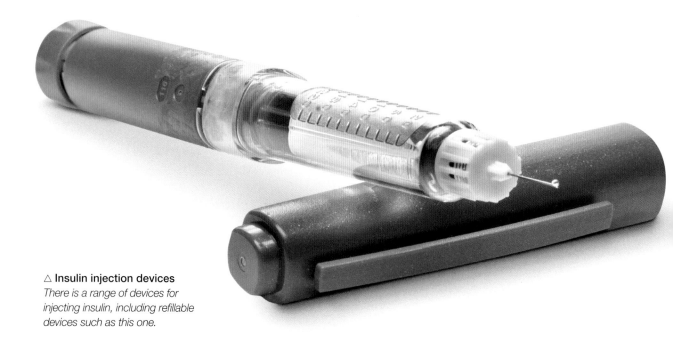

△ **Insulin injection devices**
There is a range of devices for injecting insulin, including refillable devices such as this one.

How insulin controls blood glucose

The insulin you receive by injection or pump works in the same way as the insulin produced in the pancreas of a person who doesn't have diabetes. It lowers the level of glucose in your blood by enabling your body cells to take in glucose and your liver and muscles to store glucose in the form of glycogen. Insulin also plays an important part in preventing glycogen from being converted back into glucose. This stops your blood glucose level from rising unnecessarily. Your insulin treatment aims to mimic the natural way insulin is released in your body, which is to rise and fall according to the level of glucose in your blood.

▽ **Blood glucose and insulin levels without diabetes**
The pancreas maintains a background level of insulin and produces extra when needed to deal with rises in blood glucose after eating and drinking.

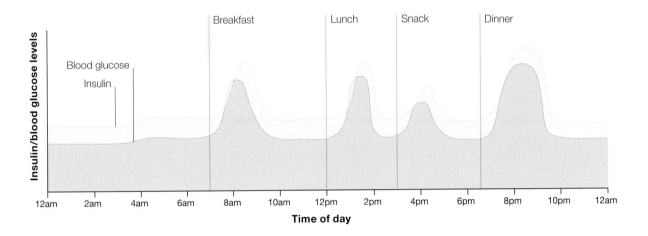

Breakfast   Lunch   Snack   Dinner

Blood glucose

Insulin

Insulin/blood glucose levels

12am   2am   4am   6am   8am   10am   12pm   2pm   4pm   6pm   8pm   10pm   12am

Time of day

Strength and dose of insulin

Insulin is measured in International Units, or "units" for short. There are 100 units to every millilitre (ml). Insulin usually comes in either a small 10 ml (1000 u) glass bottle, a 3 ml (300 u) cartridge, or a 3 ml (300 u) delivery device. Unlike other forms of medication, such as painkillers or antibiotics, there is no universal maximum or recommended dose of insulin.

Everyone's needs are different and your insulin dose will be tailored to what is right for you. You will usually start on a small dose (10–20 units per day) and increase or decrease this to keep your blood glucose level between 4–9 millimoles per litre (mmol/L) or your personalized, target range. The amount of insulin you need to keep your blood glucose level within this range will vary according to different circumstances (see pp.48–51).

Insulin dose treatment should keep blood glucose within your recommended range

▷ **Insulin units**
Insulin is measured in standard international units. A 10 ml bottle usually contains 10 ml (1000 units) of insulin. Some insulin is available as 200 units per ml.

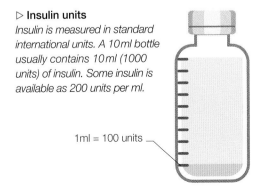

1ml = 100 units

Types of insulin

If you need insulin to manage your diabetes, you will be prescribed one or more of four main types. The difference between each type is the length of time it works in your body after injecting. You may need to change types or use different combinations from time to time.

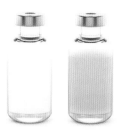

△ **Clear and cloudy**
Short- and rapid-acting insulins are always clear; intermediate-acting and pre-mixed insulins are cloudy.

Rapid-acting insulin

This clear insulin starts within minutes (see chart, opposite) so can be injected just before or up to 15 minutes before eating. It is the insulin that is used for continuous delivery (see pp.54–55). It lasts long enough to deal with the rise in blood glucose resulting from a meal, but your blood glucose level will rise once it starts to wear off. The rapid action time means that you are less likely to have a hypo (see pp.62–63) between meals.

Short-acting insulin

Also called soluble insulin, this takes 30–60 minutes to work, so you need to leave 20–30 minutes between injecting and eating. It can keep working for up to 9 hours, and you may need to balance its peak action by having a carbohydrate snack 2–3 hours after injecting to prevent your blood glucose level falling and causing a hypo. With type 1 diabetes, you also need a longer-acting insulin to ensure you have insulin available throughout the day and night.

Intermediate-acting insulin

This cloudy insulin, also called isophane insulin, helps to keep your blood glucose level in your target range throughout the day. However, you may need to eat something around its peak action time to prevent a hypo. If you have type 1 diabetes, you will be prescribed an intermediate-acting insulin with a shorter-acting insulin to stop your blood glucose level rising after your shorter-acting insulin has worn off. If you have type 2 diabetes, you may be prescribed intermediate-acting insulin in this way, or on its own, or with other types of medication (see pp.58–59).

Long-acting insulin

This clear insulin starts working within 1–2 hours and is effective for 24 hours or more. It doesn't have a peak action, so you are less likely to have a hypo than with some other insulins. If you have type 1 diabetes, you may be prescribed a long-acting insulin with rapid-acting insulin given separately to cover the rise in blood glucose at mealtimes. If you have type 2 diabetes, you may be prescribed long-acting insulin in this way, or on its own, or with tablets.

PRE-MIXED INSULINS

These ready-made combinations of rapid- or short-acting and intermediate-acting insulin come in a range of fixed proportions. Examples include biphasic insulin aspart, biphasic insulin lispro, and biphasic human isophane. They work within 30 minutes and last for 12–14 hours. Usually injected twice a day, they are useful if you want to limit injections and if you have a regular lifestyle and mealtimes.

INSULIN TYPES AND ACTION

If you have type 1 diabetes, you are most likely to be prescribed a rapid- or short-acting insulin to be taken every time you eat, along with a longer-acting insulin. If you have type 2 diabetes and need insulin, you will most likely use an intermediate- or long-acting insulin. Knowing the peak time of insulin action allows you to be aware of when you might need a carbohydrate-containing snack in order to prevent hypoglycaemia.

TYPE AND EXAMPLES	START OF ACTION	TIME OF PEAK ACTION	DURATION OF ACTION	USAGE NOTES
Rapid-acting (insulin aspart, insulin lispro)	5–15 mins	1–2 hours	2–5 hours	Prescribed for type 1 diabetes by injection or pump; often taken to cover mealtimes in combination with a longer-acting insulin. Can be used as a one-off dose.
Short-acting (soluble or neutral insulin)	30–60 mins	1–4 hours	Up to 9 hours	Prescribed for type 1 diabetes by injection. May need a carbohydrate snack around time of peak action to prevent hypoglycaemia.
Intermediate-acting (isophane insulin)	1–2 hours	3–12 hours	11–24 hours	May need a carbohydrate snack around time of peak action to prevent hypoglycaemia.
Long-acting (long-acting insulin analogues: insulin detemir, insulin glargine, insulin degludec)	1–2 hours	None	May last up to 36 hours	Provides steady background level of insulin. Prescribed for type 1 diabetes alongside rapid-acting insulin at mealtimes. For type 2 diabetes, it may be prescribed in this way, or on its own, or in combination with other types of medication.

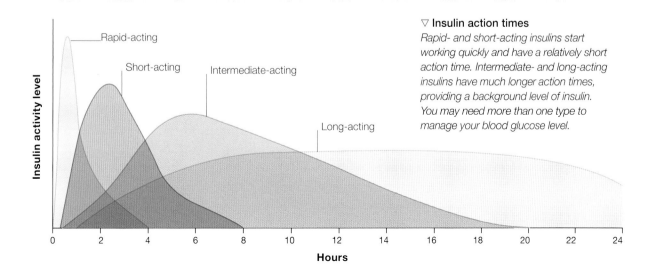

▽ **Insulin action times**
Rapid- and short-acting insulins start working quickly and have a relatively short action time. Intermediate- and long-acting insulins have much longer action times, providing a background level of insulin. You may need more than one type to manage your blood glucose level.

Insulin regimens

How often you need to have your insulin dose will depend on your type of diabetes and how well your insulin is working. The aim of the different regimens is to provide the right amount of insulin to match your blood glucose levels throughout the day.

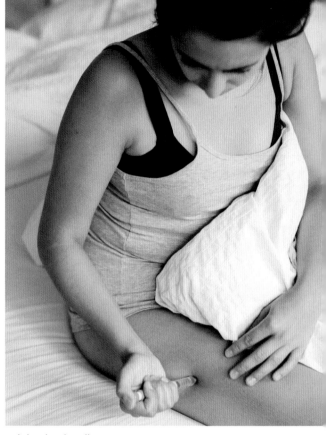

How often do I need take insulin?

If you have type 1 diabetes, you are most likely to have multiple insulin doses every day or continuous insulin through a pump. If you have type 2 diabetes, you may have insulin once or twice a day while also taking tablets.

Most people with **type 1 diabetes** have insulin **several times a day** to balance **glucose surges** at mealtimes

△ Injecting insulin
You may need to inject insulin several times a day to keep blood glucose within target range.

Multiple daily (MDI) or basal–bolus injections

This is the most likely regimen if you have type 1 diabetes. An intermediate- or long-acting insulin taken at bedtime provides a background (basal) level, while injections of rapid-acting insulin at mealtimes (bolus) deal with the surge in glucose after food. It offers flexibility about when and what you eat and helps avoid hypos. Basal insulin doses can be taken morning and evening if this helps with flexibility.

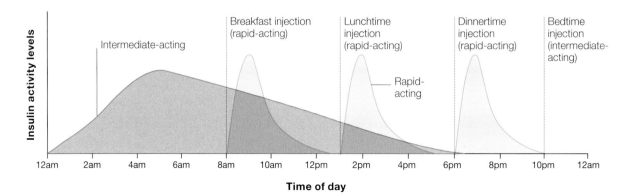

Breakfast injection (rapid-acting)

Lunchtime injection (rapid-acting)

Dinnertime injection (rapid-acting)

Bedtime injection (intermediate-acting)

Intermediate-acting

Rapid-acting

Insulin activity levels

12am 2am 4am 6am 8am 10am 12pm 2pm 4pm 6pm 8pm 10pm 12am

Time of day

Twice a day

This regimen may be used for both type 1 and type 2 diabetes. You may be prescribed an intermediate- or long-acting insulin; an intermediate-acting insulin that comes ready-mixed with a rapid- or short-acting insulin; or an intermediate-acting insulin that you mix yourself with a rapid- or short-acting insulin. An injection in the morning looks after your daytime blood glucose level. An evening injection acts on levels overnight. You need to balance this fixed regimen with meals and snacks.

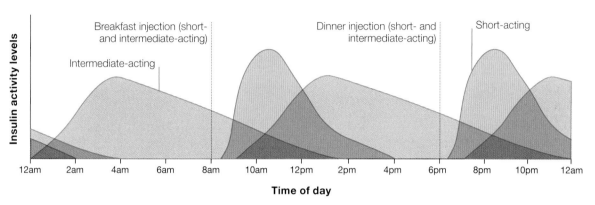

Once a day

If you have type 2 diabetes and you need to take insulin as well as other medication, you are likely to start with one injection a day to cover the rise in blood glucose that occurs before meals and in the morning. If you have type 1 diabetes, this regimen would not be suitable because it does not give you enough insulin to cover mealtimes. If the once-a-day insulin prescribed for you is a long-acting analogue, you can inject it either at bedtime or in the morning, depending on your lifestyle and to avoid hypos.

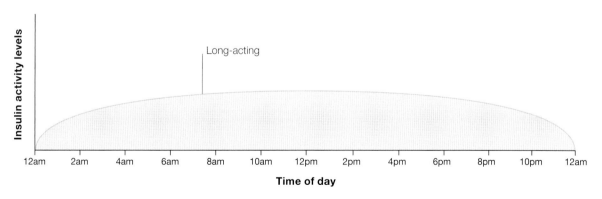

CONTINUOUS DELIVERY

Insulin pumps (see pp.54–55) provide a continuous delivery of insulin, and these are increasingly offered to people with type 1 diabetes. A pump delivers rapid-acting insulin into your body, often via a tube in your abdomen. You use the pump buttons or a remote control to deliver extra doses, called boluses, at mealtimes and when your blood glucose is high. A pump can provide a more flexible lifestyle, mainly because it gives rapid-acting insulin only, so you can quickly adjust your insulin dose to meet your needs.

Adjusting insulin doses

An important aspect of diabetes management is adjusting your dose of insulin in response to changes in your blood glucose levels. The dose of insulin you need may vary when you eat different foods, change your activity level, or are unwell or stressed.

When are changes needed?

You may need to change the number of injections you have as a result of changes in your life, such as pregnancy, illness or a new job. How often you adjust your insulin dose depends on your regimen and your blood glucose levels. You may make frequent changes, or you may only adjust your dose in special circumstances. If your blood glucose levels are often outside your target range, you may be, for example, eating more or less food than you were, or you may have changed your usual level of physical activity. You may be able to modify some aspect of your daily routine to bring your blood glucose back into range, but if not, consider adjusting your insulin dose.

It can be difficult to work out what factors may have affected your blood glucose level, and so it is useful to keep a record of key information. For example, you could record your insulin dose and blood glucose readings. You may also find it helpful to include notes that will help you to decide if you need to adjust your insulin dose. An example of a monitoring record for a multidose insulin regimen is shown on p.50; your own record may be for a range of different times rather than all of those shown. Some systems, such as continuous glucose monitors (see p.35), automatically keep a record of readings, which you can download and/or review in real time.

Adjusting a once-a-day dose

You can assess whether your insulin dose needs adjusting by checking or monitoring your blood glucose level at

If you inject insulin more than once a day, change one insulin dose at a time

KEY POINTS FOR ADJUSTING INSULIN

- Don't change your regular insulin dose in response to a single blood glucose reading.

- If your blood glucose level is high for more than a day or two, and other measures aren't working, you need more insulin.

- If your blood glucose level is low for more than a day or two, you need less insulin.

- Change only one insulin dose at a time, so that you can easily check the effect of the change through your blood glucose levels.

- Start by increasing or decreasing your insulin dose by 2–4 units at a time. If you usually take large doses of insulin, 40–60 units in a single dose for example, you may need larger dose changes to have an effect.

- If you are on a twice-a-day regimen with long-acting insulin, wait at least a day before making any further changes – this insulin stays in your body for up to 24 hours, so you need this long to assess whether your dose change has worked.

different times of the day – for example, when you get up in the morning, or before or two hours after each meal. If you change your dose and it hasn't changed your blood glucose level, consider making a further dose change in a day or two.

Adjusting a twice-a-day dose

If you take intermediate- or long-acting insulin by itself, or intermediate-acting insulin that is ready mixed with a short- or rapid-acting insulin, you need to decide which of your two injections (morning or evening) you need to adjust. If you want to influence your blood glucose level before lunch, in the afternoon, and before your evening meal, you should adjust the dose of your morning injection of insulin. If you want to influence your blood glucose level in the evening, overnight, and first thing in the morning, you should adjust the dose of your evening injection. If your changes have not improved your blood glucose level, consider making a further change.

Adjusting a multidose regimen

With a multidose regimen, you can make frequent adjustments to your dose of rapid- or short-acting insulin at mealtimes as well as changes to your longer-acting (basal) insulin. With rapid-acting insulin in particular, you can inject more or less insulin according to how much carbohydrate is in your meal (see panel, below). If you are sometimes not sure how much you are going to eat, you can inject more rapid-acting insulin after you have eaten. You can measure the effect of your insulin dose change by checking your blood glucose two hours later. If you use short-acting insulin and change the dose of your breakfast injection, this will affect your blood glucose level not just two hours after eating, but up until lunchtime because of its longer duration of action. Similarly, a change in your lunchtime dose continues to affect your blood glucose level in the late afternoon. So an increased dose might cause a hypo 4–6 hours later, even though it corrects a high blood glucose level after 2 hours.

▷ **Selecting the right dose**
You may need to adjust the amount of insulin you take at various times, according to changes in your lifestyle or when you are ill. Make sure you change the dose by gradual steps until you get the correct dose.

WORKING OUT YOUR BOLUS INSULIN DOSE

Bolus insulin is part of any basal bolus regimen. Usually, a rapid- or short-acting insulin bolus is taken before, during, or sometimes just after you have eaten. To work out how much you need, it is helpful to know your own insulin-to-carbohydrate ratio – this is the amount of insulin (in units) you need to inject for a certain amount of carbohydrate. Insulin-to-carbohydrate ratios vary, and you will have your own personal ratio that was worked out with your health professional based on factors such as your age, weight, and type of diabetes. If your insulin-to-carbohydrate ratio is 1 unit per 10 g of carbohydrate, then for a meal with 80 g of carbohydrate, you will need to take 8 units of insulin.

If your blood glucose level is raised or lowered between meals or first thing in the morning, you may need to change your longer-acting insulin dose. You will need to monitor your blood glucose several times over the day to assess the effect of any change because your insulin is working throughout this period (see p.45).

Adjusting a continuous dose

Insulin pumps (see pp.54–55) deliver rapid-acting insulin constantly. Checking your blood glucose level every 2–3 hours without eating in between and assessing how much the level fluctuates will tell you whether your insulin basal rate is set correctly. If your blood glucose

MULTIDOSE MONITORING RECORD

A record can help you decide when to adjust your insulin dose. With a multidose regimen (as in this example for type 1 diabetes), each mealtime dose can be adjusted when your blood glucose is outside your target range.

	INSULIN TAKEN : TIME AND DOSE (INTERNATIONAL UNITS)				BLOOD GLUCOSE LEVEL (mmol/L)						NOTES
	Breakfast Basal (long-acting) + rapid-acting, mixed	Lunch Rapid-acting	Dinner Rapid-acting	Bedtime Long-acting	Before breakfast	Before lunch	Mid-afternoon	Before evening meal	Before bed	Night-time	
Sun	10+6	6	8	10	5	6.2	9.6	12.3	7.6	6.8	High – Sunday lunch with pudding
Mon	10+6	6	8	10	5.3	5.8	8.8	10.2	6.5	5.5	Still high in afternoon but had no "extras" today
Tue	10+6	8	8	10	4	4.9	6.2	7	6.8	3.2	Night-time hypo – not sure why
Wed	10+6	8	8	8	3.8	5.2	5.8	6.2	6.4	5.6	Lower BG in the night and early morning so reduced night-time basal dose
Thu	10+6	8	8	8	4.8	3.6	10.3	7.1	5.8	6.2	Better overnight but hypo at lunchtime and rebound high (due to morning aerobics)
Fri	10+4	8	8	8	6.3	5.7	6.4	5.8	6.5	6.5	Reduced morning rapid as walking to work – no hypo
Sat	10+6	6	6	6	7.2	6.3	8.6	7.5	8.0	5.4	Less insulin because drinking in afternoon and evening – seemed to work well

rises or falls more than 1–2 millimoles per litre (mmol/L), you can increase or reduce your insulin dose to prevent this from happening.

Dealing with different situations

Various situations commonly cause changes in blood glucose and when you are likely to need to make adjustments to your insulin.

Eating out

If you are eating out or might eat more than usual, you can prevent your blood glucose rising above your target by increasing your insulin dose before you eat. Alternatively, if you use rapid-acting insulin, you can take extra insulin after you have eaten, basing the dose on the type and size of your meal. When you increase your insulin dose, work out how long the insulin will stay in your body and when it will have its peak effect (see p.45) because you may need to have a snack at this point to avoid hypoglycaemia.

Physical activity

Your blood glucose may fall in response to physical activity (see pp.104–107). If you are going to be more active than usual, you may need to lower your insulin dose to avoid a hypo.

Illness

A rise in blood glucose is a normal part of your body's response to illness, even if you are not eating. It can slow your recovery time as well as increase the risk of diabetic ketoacidosis (see p.71) if you have type 1 diabetes, or hyperosmolar hyperglycaemic state (see p.71) if you have type 2 diabetes. It is important to increase your insulin dose, based on

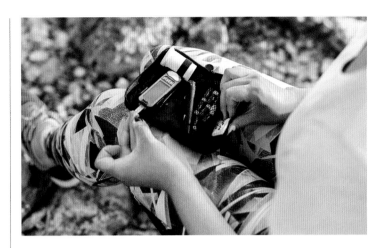

frequent blood glucose readings, to keep your glucose level at least below 10 mmol/L. During illness, this increase may be 2–4 units or more at each dose. Alternatively, your health professional may recommend more frequent insulin. As you recover, your blood glucose level usually falls and you will need to reduce your insulin again.

Fasting

If you are otherwise well and fasting, you will need to reduce your insulin dose. With type 1 diabetes, you need a lower-than-usual dose throughout the fast. If you have type 2 diabetes, you may be able to have a much reduced insulin dose or even stop it altogether while you are fasting (your body may still be able to produce some insulin itself).

If you are not fasting completely but are giving up some types of food, you need to tailor your insulin regimen so that you receive enough insulin when you eat but not so much that you become hypoglycaemic at other times. A basal-bolus regimen using a rapid-acting insulin may be useful. Discuss the options with your health professional.

△ **Mid-exercise glucose checks**
By checking your blood glucose before and after exercise, you can work out whether or not you need a change to your insulin.

Insulin equipment and care

There is a wide variety of equipment designed to deliver insulin. The most widely used are pen devices. Insulin pumps are increasingly popular as they make managing your insulin doses more flexible. However, the traditional needle and syringe is still useful, especially as a back-up. Another important item is a sharps box, to dispose of used equipment safely.

Injection devices

The injection equipment you are offered depends on the type and brand of insulin you are taking, as well as your insulin regimen and dose. Devices for children are similar to those for adults but usually have a more child-friendly appearance.

Pen-shaped devices

There are many different pen-shaped insulin devices – the main difference is whether they are reusable or disposable.

With a reusable device, you take the device apart to insert a cartridge of insulin (which typically contains 300 units) into a holder. You then reassemble the device,

attach a needle, do an air shot, then dial your dose of insulin (see p.57). When you have used all the insulin in the cartridge, you insert a new one. A reusable pen can last many years.

Other reusable devices include jet injectors, which fire a stream of insulin from a cartridge through your skin without using a needle. Many resusable devices include a log of the time and amount of your last dose of insulin, or you can add a separate logging device to record this information (see p.54).

Disposable devices are similar to resusable ones but have a cartridge of insulin already inside. You use a

REUSABLE PEN

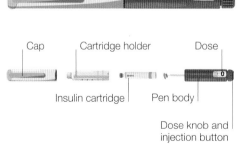

△ **Reusable pen devices**
These have a replaceable insulin cartridge, which is inserted into a holder. When the cartridge is empty, you replace it with a new one.

DISPOSABLE PEN

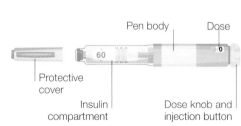

△ **Disposable pen device**
Disposable devices are prefilled with insulin; once the insulin has been used, the entire device is thrown away.

disposable device in the same way as a reusable one, except that when it is empty, you dispose of the entire device. Disposable devices may last for a few days or several weeks, depending on how much insulin you take.

Dial-up devices

These are disposable devices that have a large dosage dial on the front, so that it is easy to see the dose you are setting. They are usually prefilled with 300 units of insulin. They also have single-use needles, and a plunger that you press to inject.

Syringes

A traditional syringe consists of a plastic tube with insulin units marked on the outside and a fixed needle. You use it to draw up insulin from a bottle (see p.56). Traditional syringes are small and light, which makes them easy to carry around with you, although filling them may be less convenient or discreet if you are out. They are available in different sizes to accommodate different dosages, and with different needle lengths.

SYRINGE

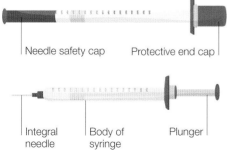

Needle safety cap   Protective end cap

Integral   Body of   Plunger
needle   syringe

△ **Traditional syringes**
These come fitted with a needle and are disposed of after a single use. They have numbers on the body to show insulin units.

NEEDLES

These attach to your injection device and must be replaced after each single use. The are available in various sizes, from 4 mm to 12.7 mm long. You will usually be offered the smallest size first, but may need to use a larger size if you experience bruising or leaking.

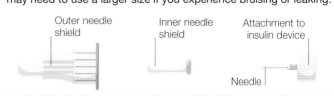

Outer needle shield   Inner needle shield   Attachment to insulin device

Needle

Injection aids

If you want to distract yourself while injecting, limit the number of times you inject, or have trouble keeping track of the doses you have taken, various devices are available to help.

Distraction aids

An injection distraction aid can hide the needle of an injection device or brush against the skin while the injection is being given to distract your attention.

Port device

A port device consists of a short cannula (hollow tube) attached to a cover with a small hole to accommodate a needle. The cannula is inserted into the skin. When you want to inject, you insert the needle into the

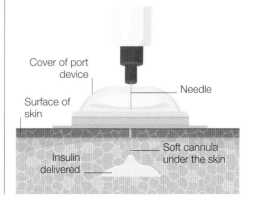

Cover of port device

Surface of skin

Needle

Insulin delivered

Soft cannula under the skin

◁ **Port device**
A port device is inserted into the skin and can remain in place for several days. The cover has an adhesive so that it remains firmly attached to the skin.

Display

Connection for infusion tube

Operating buttons

Infusion set

Attachment to pump

Tubing

Insulin reservoir

INSULIN PUMP

CONNECTION TO SKIN

◁ **Tethered insulin pump**
This type of pump has simple controls and a display screen. A refillable cartridge contains your insulin. A small plastic tube is attached to the pump at one end and to the infusion set at the other. The infusion set consists of a hollow needle (cannula) inserted under the skin and an adhesive cover.

hole and administer your dose of insulin. The insulin then travels down the cannula into your body. This device is useful for giving multiple daily doses of insulin without needing to puncture the skin each time. Instead, you change the port device every few days.

Dosage logs
These are devices that replace the protective needle cover of your pen device and automatically record the time since your previous insulin dose. More sophisticated versions can also record the amount and type of insulin, and some can link to a smartphone or mobile device to download the results, making it easier to keep track of your insulin doses.

Insulin pumps
An Insulin pump is a small, battery-operated device with a reservoir that you fill with insulin; instead of a reservoir, some types accept cartridges of insulin. The pump delivers insulin either directly into you body (a patch pump) or via a fine tube connected to your abdomen through a small needle (cannula) under your skin (a tethered pump). You change the tubing and the cannula every few days. You can programme the pump to deliver continuous background (basal) insulin then give an extra dose (bolus) of insulin whenever you eat, or if your glucose level rises above your target range.

A pump will record your insulin doses and will sound an alarm if it is not working properly or if its insulin supply is running out. It will also help you calculate your bolus doses. A pump is worn continuously. You can keep the pump section of a tethered pump in your pocket or attached to your belt or clothes. However, you can remove it for short periods (up to about an hour), for example, for swimming or showering.

Adjusting your insulin dose with a pump
Insulin pumps have extensive menus, so you can choose the one that suits your needs. For example, if you know you will be snacking throughout a celebration or an evening out, you can set an extended bolus to prevent your blood glucose from rising above your target level. Similarly, you can reduce your basal delivery rate for when you know you will be more active than usual. Some pumps are able to suspend your insulin delivery if you are at risk of a hypo. Many pumps can be programmed using an app on a smartphone or other mobile device.

Use with a continuous glucose meter
Most insulin pumps are compatible with a continuous glucose monitor (CGM, see p.35 and p.37).The CGM reads your blood glucose level all the time and sends the information to the pump and also to a separate device, which you can use to

PROS AND CONS OF INSULIN PUMPS

Deciding whether an insulin pump is right for you is an important step. Pumps have both advantages and disadvantages, and it can be helpful to talk with your health professional before making a decision. It may also be possible to trial one first to see if it benefits you.

PROS	CONS
No need for multiple injections; only need to change cannula every 2–3 days.	Feeling "attached" to your diabetes all the time.
Flexibility – for example, over meal times and physical activity.	Having to respond to alarms or prompts.
More accurately able to match insulin to different foods and activities.	Rare risk of pump malfunctioning or accidentally breaking.
Can take immediate action if blood glucose is too high or too low, and see the effect quckly.	Explaining and responding to security staff if they are not familiar with or are suspicious of the pump.
Feeling more in charge of your diabetes.	If using a CGM or flash monitor, needing to wear a number of devices, and also needing to do regular fingerprick blood glucose checks.

adjust your insulin dose. Some pumps automatically adjust basal insulin delivery every few minutes, based on the CGM readings. This helps avoid blood glucose highs and lows.

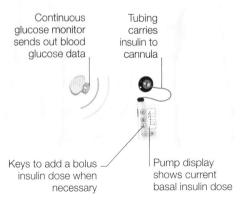

Continuous glucose monitor sends out blood glucose data

Tubing carries insulin to cannula

Keys to add a bolus insulin dose when necessary

Pump display shows current basal insulin dose

△ **Continuous monitor linked with pump**
A CGM reads blood glucose levels and sends this information to the pump and also to a remote device. Some pumps can adjust the basal insulin dose in response to this information. The remote device can also be used to adjust the insulin dose.

Storage, care, and disposal

All your equipment and supplies need to be stored, used, and replaced according to the manufacturer's recommendations. In particular, it is important to use a new needle for each injection or a new disposable syringe, and to replace pump tubing regularly.

Unopened insulin needs to be kept in a fridge at 2–8°C. The insulin you are using can be kept out of the fridge for up to a month at temperatures of up to 25°C, provided it is kept out of direct sunlight. If it is hotter than this, you will need to keep it cool. From time to time, it is wise to check that your insulin supplies are within their "use by" date.

Used or out-of-date equipment should be disposed of safely. Needles, disposable syringes, and any items with blood on should be put in a special sharps box. Your health professional will advise you about safe disposal of the box.

Injecting insulin

Preparing your insulin and using the correct technique to inject is important for insulin to work effectively. The precise process of injecting yourself depends on whether you are using an insulin device (see opposite), or a syringe (see below). You need to change your injection site each time.

> **PREPARING TO INJECT**
>
> - Check your insulin's appearance and expiry date. If it's cloudy when it's meant to be clear, has a pink tinge, looks lumpy, or contains particles even after gentle rotation, discard it and use a new bottle, cartridge, or disposable device.
> - Make sure you have everything ready that you need: insulin device and new needle; a sharps bin or needle clipper; and cotton wool or tissue in case of any bleeding.

Choosing your injection site

Insulin is injected into the fat layer just under your skin. Several factors might influence which site you inject. Insulin can work more quickly if injected into the abdomen rather than the buttocks, for example. It also works faster if injected just before any exercise that uses that part of the body (for example, the thigh before cycling). If using rapid- or short-acting insulin, injecting into the abdomen works well. With premixed insulin, it's effective to inject into the abdomen in the morning and thighs or buttocks in the evening. You need to rotate injection sites regularly to avoid problems with absorption due to lipohypertrophy (see p.198).

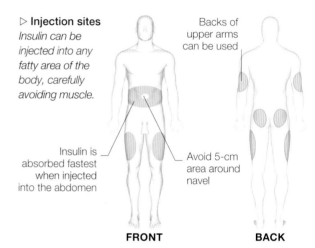

▷ **Injection sites**
Insulin can be injected into any fatty area of the body, carefully avoiding muscle.

Backs of upper arms can be used

Insulin is absorbed fastest when injected into the abdomen

Avoid 5-cm area around navel

FRONT   **BACK**

USING A SYRINGE

Check the appearance and expiry date of your insulin and gently invert the bottle to resuspend the insulin if it's cloudy. Ensure that the top of the insulin bottle is clean, and use a new syringe each time you inject. After you have injected, clip the needle and dispose of the syringe safely.

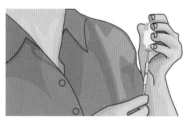

1 Draw air into the syringe to match the insulin needed. Insert the needle into the bottle. Invert and check that the tip of the needle is in the insulin.

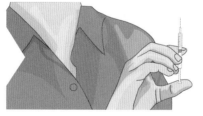

2 Pull the plunger back to draw up insulin. When you have the correct dose, withdraw the needle. With the syringe upright, flick it and then gently press the plunger to remove any air bubbles.

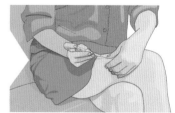

3 Check you have the correct amount, insert the needle (using the pinch-up technique if advised), and press the plunger. Hold for a count of 10 before removing.

USING AN INSULIN DEVICE

Most insulin-injecting devices work in the same way, although the details may vary slightly from one device to another – consult the manufacturer's instructions if you are in any doubt. Check the appearance and expiry date of your insulin before you inject. Wash your hands and ensure you have everything you need (see opposite). After you have finished, dispose of the needle as advised by your health professional.

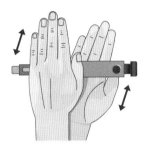

1 Pull off the outer cover of the device. If you are using premixed or cloudy insulin, roll the device between your hands 10 times.

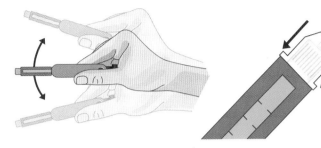

2 After rolling the device, gently invert it 10 times. (This and the preceding step are not needed for clear insulin.)

3 Take a new needle and push it on to the device, ensuring the needle is in line with the device and properly attached.

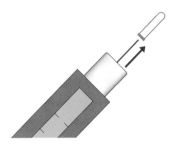

4 Twist the needle in place, then remove the outer cap and inner cap to expose the needle.

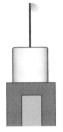

5 Holding the device upright, dial a small dose (2–4 units) and press the plunger until a drop of insulin appears at the end of the needle.

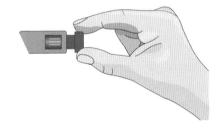

6 You are now ready to dial the dose that you need to inject.

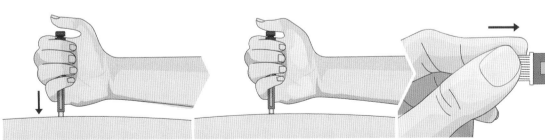

7 Position the device at an angle of 90 degrees to your body.

8 Press the plunger, keeping it depressed to inject your dose of insulin. Ensure the dial goes back to 0, and leave in place for 10 seconds.

9 After removing the device, dispose of the needle as advised by your health professional. Replace the device's outer cover.

Other diabetes medication

If you have type 2 diabetes, you are most likely to be treated with non-insulin medication, which may be taken as tablets or injections. There are many types, all of which work to manage your blood glucose levels so that you stay healthy long-term.

The right medication

Diabetes tablets work in various ways to help keep blood glucose levels within the recommended range in type 2 diabetes (see chart, opposite). For example, some stimulate your pancreas to produce more insulin; others slow down glucose entering your bloodstream; and some enable your body cells to take up insulin better.

Your health professional will take into account different factors when deciding which medication to recommend for you, including your weight, lifestyle, and blood glucose level. If you are overweight, then drugs that cause weight gain won't be the first choice. If your eating pattern is irregular, then a drug that has a short duration of action will be better than a longer-acting one. Medication is initially prescribed on a trial basis to see how well it suits you and to assess its effectiveness. You will have an HbA1c check (see p.31) after 3 months to see how well your medication is working. If your HbA1c level remains outside your target range, the dose may be increased or another medication added.

You may need to try more than one medication, or different combinations, before you find what works best for you

> ### REMEMBERING TO TAKE YOUR MEDICATION
>
> - Every morning, count out your medication for the day, and check you have taken it all at the end of the day.
> - Put the medication in a place that will remind you to take it.
> - Prepare your medication at the same time you get your meal ready.
> - If necessary, set an alert or alarm on your mobile phone, computer, or other device to remind you to take your medication.
> - If possible, ask someone to remind you at the time you need to take your medication.
> - Keep a supply of medication with you so that you can take it wherever you are.

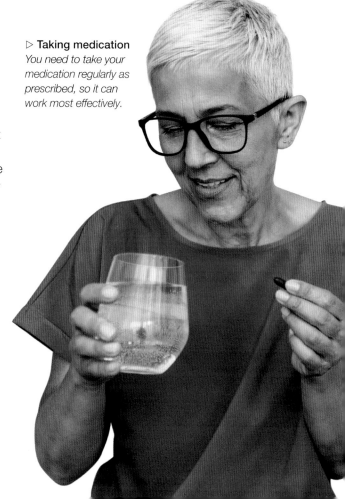

▷ **Taking medication**
You need to take your medication regularly as prescribed, so it can work most effectively.

MEDICATIONS FOR TYPE 2 DIABETES

Different medications have different actions, doses, and side effects. Speak to your health professional if you have any concerns about the medication you take. Most drugs are not recommended if you are pregnant or breastfeeding. Never exceed the daily dose or stop taking your medication without consulting your health professional first.

MEDICATION TYPE AND ACTION	EXAMPLES	HOW TAKEN AND WHEN TO TAKE	POSSIBLE SIDE EFFECTS
Sulphonylureas Increase the amount of insulin the pancreas produces; also increase the effectiveness of insulin	Glibenclamide, gliclazide, glipizide, glimepiride, tolbutamide	Tablets; taken once or twice a day, with or shortly before a meal	Weight gain; hypos
Prandial glucose regulators (meglitinides) Similar to sulphonylureas, increase the amount of insulin the pancreas produces	Nateglinide, repaglinide	Tablets; taken within 30 minutes of starting a meal	Weight gain; hypos. Side effects less frequent than those produced by sulphonylureas
Biguanides Increase the body cells' sensitivity to insulin; also reduce glucose production by the liver	Metformin immediate release	Tablets; taken two to three times a day with or after food	Nausea; diarrhoea; abdominal pain
	Metformin prolonged release	Tablets; taken once a day with or after food	
Alpha glucosidase inhibitors Slow down the digestion of carbohydrates in starchy foods, which slows glucose entering bloodstream	Acarbose	Tablets; taken at the start of, or immediately before, a meal	Flatulence; diarrhoea
Glitazones (thiazolidinediones) Reduce body cells' resistance to insulin so help cells to take up insulin better	Pioglitazone	Tablets; taken once or twice a day, with or without food	Visual disturbance; weight gain; fluid retention; increased risk of bone fractures
Gliptins (DPP-4 inhibitors) Increase insulin release from pancreas; slow down digestion and decrease appetite; lower blood glucose levels	Sitagliptin, vildagliptin, saxagliptin, alogliptin, linagliptin	Tablets; taken once or twice a day, with or without food	Rash; upper respiratory infections; headache; nausea
Gliflozins (SGLT2 inhibitors) Cause kidneys to excrete excess glucose into the urine	Dapagliflozin, canagliflozin, empagliflozin	Tablets; taken once a day, with or without food	Urinary tract infections; thrush (yeast infection); genital tract infections and itching
Incretin mimetics (GLP-1 analogues) Increase insulin release from pancreas in response to food and reduce glucose production by liver	Exenatide, liraglutide, lixisenatide, dulaglutide	By injection; once or twice a day or once a week, depending on the specific medication	Nausea and/or vomiting, which are often short-lived

Advances in treatment

Diabetes is the focus of a great deal of research into potential new treatments, although it may take many years for some to become available. Recent or near-future developments include new forms of insulin, immunotherapy, islet cell transplants, and new technology.

New forms of insulin

The types of insulin currently available work in your body for a certain length of time, regardless of your blood glucose level. Researchers are trying to develop a new form of insulin, known as glucose-responsive or "smart" insulin, that automatically responds to your blood glucose level to keep it within the recommended range. Although smart insulin is still in its experimental stages, if it proves successful it would make it much easier to manage your blood glucose level.

Immunotherapy for type 1 diabetes

Modifying the activity of the immune system with medication – known as immunotherapy – is already being used successfully to treat rheumatoid arthritis and other autoimmune conditions in which the immune system mistakenly destroys certain body cells. Similar drug treatments are being developed for type 1 diabetes – also an autoimmune condition – with the aim of preventing the immune system from destroying the insulin-producing islet cells in the pancreas. If these new drugs prove to be effective, they could be used to delay or prevent the onset of type 1 diabetes in people who have been identified by genetic testing to be at risk of developing the condition but have not yet done so.

Islet cell transplants

The aim of an islet cell transplant is to introduce healthy, insulin-producing islet cells into a person with type 1 diabetes, whose own islet cells have been destroyed. The procedure usually works well in reducing severe hypos and improving the quality of life of recipients. However, they need to take anti-rejection medication for the rest of their lives, and this can produce side effects. In addition,

Transplanting islet cells

An islet cell transplant involves removing pancreas tissue from the donor organ, separating out the insulin-producing islet cells, and then transferring the cells to a recipient with type 1 diabetes.

DONOR

1 **Pancreas tissue removed**
A sample of pancreas tissue containing islet cells is removed from a deceased donor who has given consent for their organs to be used for transplantation.

Pancreas contains islet cells that produce insulin

Pancreas

Pancreas tissue removed from donor

many recipients still need to take some insulin after a transplant, although their insulin requirements are usually lower. Not everybody is suitable for a transplant, and the number that can be performed is limited by the relatively small number of donor pancreases available.

New technology

Advances in technology are helping to make diabetes management easier and more precise. For example, smart pen devices (not yet available worldwide) store data that you can download later, which means that you can easily record dates, times, and amounts of your insulin doses, carbohydrate intake, and blood glucose levels. An advance that seems likely to become more widely available in the

near future is the closed loop or artificial pancreas system, consisting of an insulin pump, a continuous glucose monitor, and a communication link. The monitor sends data to a small computer, which uses an algorithm to instruct the pump to adjust your insulin dose according to your blood glucose level. The system displays on your smartphone or smartwatch, and you can also revert to manual control.

TAKING PART IN RESEARCH

Research may range from simply completing a questionnaire to something more involved, such as trying new therapies. Official research requires formal consent, so that you are fully informed and can withdraw at any time. If you are interested in participating, your diabetes healthcare professionals or diabetes organizations will be able to provide up-to-date information.

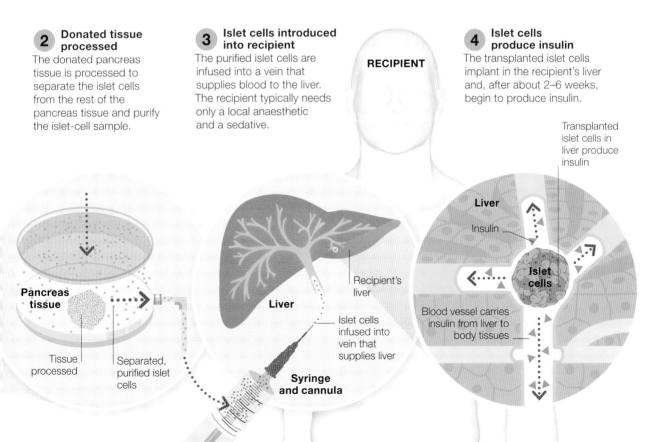

2 **Donated tissue processed**

The donated pancreas tissue is processed to separate the islet cells from the rest of the pancreas tissue and purify the islet-cell sample.

3 **Islet cells introduced into recipient**

The purified islet cells are infused into a vein that supplies blood to the liver. The recipient typically needs only a local anaesthetic and a sedative.

RECIPIENT

4 **Islet cells produce insulin**

The transplanted islet cells implant in the recipient's liver and, after about 2–6 weeks, begin to produce insulin.

Transplanted islet cells in liver produce insulin

Pancreas tissue

Tissue processed

Separated, purified islet cells

Liver

Recipient's liver

Islet cells infused into vein that supplies liver

Syringe and cannula

Liver

Insulin

Islet cells

Blood vessel carries insulin from liver to body tissues

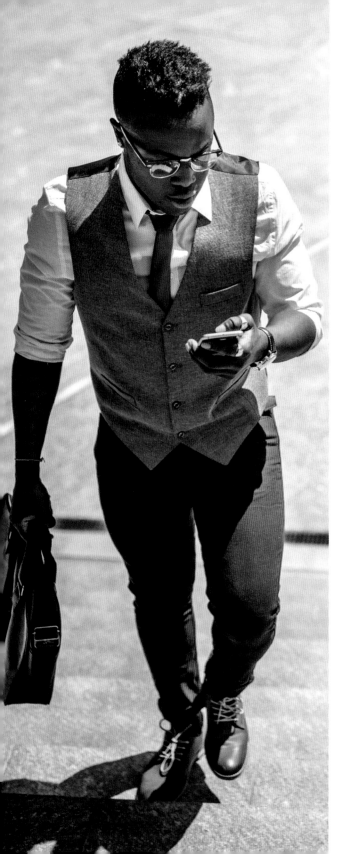

Hypoglycaemia

Commonly known as a "hypo", hypoglycaemia is when your blood glucose level falls too low. It is often due to a dose of insulin or insulin-stimulating medication that is too high in relation to your food intake. Being aware of factors that trigger a hypo can help you to prevent one.

What is hypoglycaemia?

In practical terms, a hypo means a blood glucose level below 4 millimoles per litre (mmol/L). Hypos occur when there is more insulin in your body than you need at the time, typically because your insulin or medication dose does not match your food intake or level of activity. Hypos often cause recognizable symptoms (see pp.64–65), although the blood glucose level at which symptoms become noticeable can vary from person to person, and symptoms may be more pronounced in some people than others.

◁ **Fitting in food**
A busy lifestyle can make it difficult to eat regularly. However, missing or delaying eating puts you at risk of a hypo, so it is helpful to be aware of when to eat and to set up reminders for yourself.

PREVENTING AND ACTING ON HYPOS

- Keep checking your blood glucose several hours after vigorous activity as delayed hypos can occur.

- If it helps to involve others, ask your family, friends, or colleagues to remind you to check your blood glucose and to eat snacks regularly.

- Keep glucose and carbohydrate snacks handy.

- If you have frequent hypos, talk to your health professional about changing your medication type or timing to better suit your routine.

CAUSES AND PREVENTION

Various factors may trigger a hypo; the more common ones are detailed in this chart. It is important to try to prevent hypos and treat them promptly (see pp.66–67) before your blood glucose drops too low, because a very low level can make you feel unwell, stop you thinking clearly, and even, in some situations, cause you to lose consciousness.

CAUSE	PREVENTION
Medication dose	If you take insulin, an occasional hypo is to be expected. You are also at risk of hypos if you take insulin-stimulating medications (see pp.58–59). Other diabetes medications taken on their own do not carry a significant hypo risk.	If you have hypos frequently, you may need a lower dose of insulin or medication. If you take insulin or other medication several times a day, it is important to identify which injection or tablet is responsible for the hypo and then adjust that dose.
Food intake	Injected insulin and insulin-stimulating medication work over a number of hours, and if you do not eat during this period, you risk having a hypo.	If you use insulin or insulin-stimulating medication, you need to know whether it has a peak of action, and if so, when this is so that you can balance your insulin dose or medication with carbohydrate-containing foods. If you are unsure about the timing of food for your particular insulin or medication regimen, talk it through with your health professional.
Alcohol	Initially, alcohol causes your blood glucose to rise but then, over a period of hours, causes it to fall, putting you at risk of a hypo if you take insulin or insulin-stimulating medication. Hypos due to drinking are particularly dangerous and in some circumstances can be life-threatening, because alcohol prevents your liver from releasing stored glucose efficiently.	You can prevent an alcohol-induced or prolonged hypo by never drinking on an empty stomach and, if you drink more than 2–3 units of alcohol, by eating extra carbohydrate to compensate. Checking your blood glucose after drinking (or asking somebody to help you with this) is also important.
Physical activity	Any sort of physical activity – including everyday tasks, such as housework or shopping – needs energy, which is mainly obtained from glucose. The more active you are, the more glucose you "burn" and the more your blood glucose falls.	You can prevent a hypo by reducing the dose of your insulin or insulin-stimulating medication before any physical activity or by eating extra food before, during, or after activity. Prolonged or strenuous activity requires more careful planning (see pp.100–107).
Stress	Stress usually makes your blood glucose rise due to the effects of the stress hormones adrenaline and cortisol. However, in some people or situations, stress may make your blood glucose fall because your body may use extra energy when you are stressed, or you may not eat regularly.	Try to establish what effect stress has on your blood glucose. If you know that it lowers your blood glucose, you can compensate by eating extra food or reducing your dose of insulin or insulin-stimulating medication.
Heat	Exposure to heat makes your blood circulate more quickly, which means that insulin and insulin-stimulating medication work faster than usual. This, in turn, causes your blood glucose to fall. You may find that you are prone to hypos in hot conditions, even after a hot bath or sauna.	Checking your blood glucose before exposing yourself to unusual heat will help you identify if you are close to a hypo and whether you need extra food to avoid one. In similar situations in the future, you may need to reduce your dose of insulin or insulin-stimulating medication or eat extra food.

Recognizing hypoglycaemia

A low level of glucose in the blood – hypoglycaemia – is potentially serious but recognizing the symptoms as soon as possible usually enables the condition to be treated quickly and easily. The symptoms are more pronounced in some people than others, and if you are not able to detect your own symptoms, you may need to rely on people around you for help.

Early warning symptoms

When your blood glucose first starts to fall, you may experience early symptoms of a hypo (see table, opposite), because your body releases adrenaline in an attempt to raise your blood glucose. You may not have all or even any of these symptoms. It is also possible to experience early symptoms due to any rapid fall in blood glucose – for example, from 15 millimoles per litre (mmol/L) to 7 mmol/L. Checking your blood glucose level will give you the data to decide if any action is necessary. A fingerprick check gives a "snapshot" reading but does not reveal whether your blood glucose level is changing. In contrast, a continuous monitor or flash monitor shows your glucose level and whether it is rising, falling, or constant. If you have symptoms and your test result is 4 mmol/L or lower, you should start to treat yourself immediately (see pp.66–67).

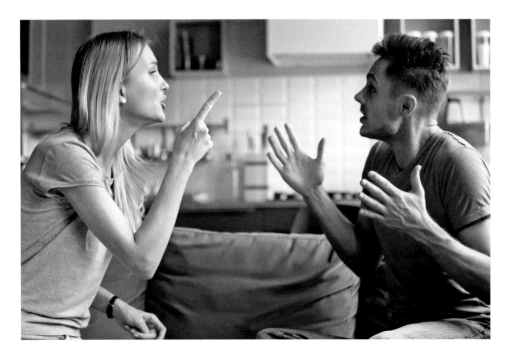

◁ **Uncharacteristic behaviour**
A hypo can affect the way you behave, for example, by making you anxious, tearful, irritable, or uncooperative.

EARLIER HYPO SYMPTOMS		LATER HYPO SYMPTOMS
Anxiety	Trembling	Headache; difficulty in concentrating; disorientation; being uncooperative and/or aggressive
Dilated pupils	Palpitations; fast pulse	Blurred vision
Skin turns paler; sweating	Hunger	Slurred speech
Tingling of lips	Nausea	Unsteady movements

Later symptoms

When your blood glucose falls below about 3 mmol/L, your brain does not receive enough glucose to function properly. As a result, many of the later symptoms of a hypo affect mental functioning. Sometimes, you may know that you are having a hypo but may not be able to think clearly enough to treat yourself and may need help. Your family members, friends, and colleagues can become skilled at recognizing a hypo and giving you or encouraging you to accept treatment. Without treatment, you may have a seizure or lose consciousness if your blood glucose continues to fall.

Reduced awareness of symptoms

Over a long period of time, or if you have a period of frequent hypos, your body can become less efficient at giving early warnings. If you have had diabetes for years and have often had hypos, you may not have any warning signs at all and your only symptoms may be confusion and disorientation. Without help, you may lose consciousness. If you do experience frequent hypos and reduced awareness of symptoms, your health professional may suggest, for example, that you temporarily allow your blood glucose to rise above the ideal range of 4–9 mmol/L to give you a respite from hypos and help restore your awareness of symptoms.

A hypo may not always produce warning symptoms

CONTINUOUS BLOOD GLUCOSE MONITORS AND FLASH MONITORS

These types of monitors display both your blood glucose level and its direction. Some continuous monitors can also be set up to sound an alarm when you are heading for a hypo, so that you can take action to prevent it. You will need to confirm a hypo with a fingerprick check, because there is a short time lag between your true blood glucose level and the reading shown by a continuous or flash monitor.

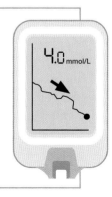

Treating hypoglycaemia

It is usually possible to treat a hypo yourself if you recognize the symptoms early. However, if a hypo becomes more severe, you may need help. In some situations, a hypo may need emergency medical treatment.

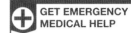

GET EMERGENCY MEDICAL HELP

- If your usual treatment isn't working and you continue to be hypoglycaemic.
- If a person having a hypo has been drinking alcohol.
- If a person having a hypo has a seizure.
- If a person having a hypo becomes unconscious and there is nobody to inject glucagon or a glucagon kit is not available.

Treating early hypoglycaemia

As soon as you realize that you are having a hypo, you must eat or drink something sugary immediately to raise your blood glucose: the panel (below right) gives some suitable examples. Any of these will raise your blood glucose within about 10–15 minutes and you will usually begin to recover. Afterwards, you need to eat something more substantial that contains carbohydrate, such as a sandwich, piece of fruit, or bowl of cereal. The exact amount you need to eat depends on the circumstances. For example, you will need to eat more if you won't be eating again for some time, whereas if you have a hypo just before a meal containing carbohydrate, the meal may be enough for you to recover fully.

Treating advanced hypoglycaemia

If you are already in the later stages of a hypo, you may be confused, losing consciousness, or unconscious. In this situation, it is dangerous to eat or drink anything. Instead, you need an injection of glucagon (a hormone that causes glucose to be released from your liver into your bloodstream) or glucose to quickly raise your blood glucose level.

To be prepared for this possibility, your health professional will prescribe you glucagon, and they can show a friend or relative how to inject it. If there is nobody available who knows how to give you glucagon, you will need medical help.

You can **treat a hypo** in its early stages by **eating or drinking** something high in **sugar**

RAISING YOUR BLOOD GLUCOSE QUICKLY

Immediately you notice symptoms of a hypo, you need to raise your blood glucose quickly to prevent it from getting worse. You can do this by eating or drinking a fast-acting carbohydrate. This could be:

 3 glucose or dextrose tablets

 5 jelly babies or jelly beans

 A small glass (120–200ml) of sugary soft drink (non-diet)

 A small carton (200ml) of pure fruit juice

 2 tubes of glucose or dextrose gel

TREATING A HYPO IN AN UNCONSCIOUS PERSON

If a hypo causes unconsciousness, you will need to give the person a glucagon injection, if you have been trained how to do so. If a glucagon injection kit is not available or you have not been shown how to inject, you need to get emergency medical help.

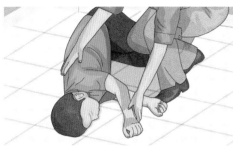

1 Put the person in the recovery position: on their side, with their arm and upper leg at right angles to their body, and their head tilted back to keep the airway clear.

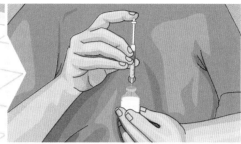

2 If you have a glucagon injection kit, remove the seal on the glucagon bottle. Uncap the needle, put it into the bottle, and inject the water from the syringe into the bottle.

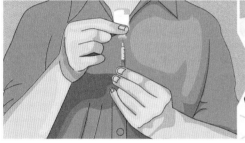

3 Rotate the bottle until all the glucagon has dissolved. Turn the bottle upside down and put the needle tip in the solution. Pull back the plunger to withdraw all the solution or the dose you have been prescribed.

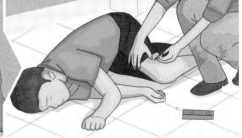

4 Insert the needle at a right angle to the person's thigh, buttock, or arm, and press the plunger to inject. Withdraw the needle, press a tissue/swab against the injection site, and keep the person in the recovery position until they are conscious.

The recovery period

If you don't receive treatment for a hypo, and even if you lose consciousness, eventually your body will naturally raise your blood glucose if the hypo is not too severe. However, if you have a very large amount of insulin and/or alcohol in your blood, your hypo will last longer and could be life-threatening; in this situation, you will need emergency medical help. During the recovery period, your blood glucose may rise too high (rebound hyperglycaemia). This may happen soon after a hypo or during the following 24 hours. If you take rapid-acting insulin, a small dose can correct rebound hyperglycaemia, but increasing the dose of other insulins may cause further hypos. Instead, try to work out the cause of the hypo in order to prevent a recurrence (see pp.62–63).

Hyperglycaemia

A blood glucose level that is too high is known as hyperglycaemia. It is the main effect of untreated diabetes. Your diabetes treatment is aimed at reducing hyperglycaemia while also avoiding hypoglycaemia (low blood glucose, see pp.62–63).

What is hyperglycaemia?

This is the technical term for blood glucose levels above about 7 millimoles per litre (mmol/L). Hyperglycaemia may not only make you feel unwell in the short term, but also increases your risk of long-term complications. This is why a blood glucose level of 4–9 mmol/L is recommended, depending on your age and the type of diabetes you have (see p.30 and p.38). However, in daily life with diabetes, you will sometimes experience periods of hyperglycaemia, and taking action to prevent them (see opposite) or limit their length (see pp.70–71) will help to keep you well.

GENERAL PREVENTIVE MEASURES

- If you know you are going to eat more carbohydrates than usual, adjust your insulin or medication, or be more active.

- Be aware of the effect of stress and other hormonal changes on your blood glucose so you can predict when you need to adjust your treatment.

- Don't stop taking your insulin or other medication when you are ill, and monitor your blood glucose frequently.

- Take your insulin or medication every day, and adjust the dose when necessary.

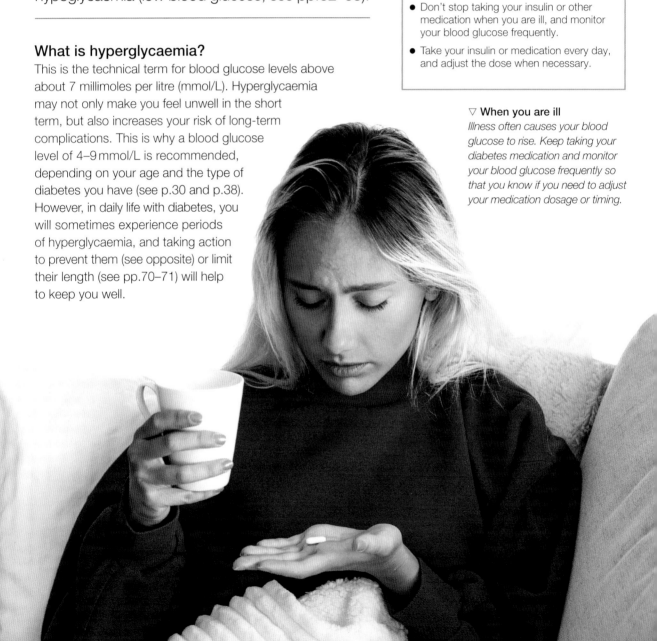

▽ **When you are ill**
Illness often causes your blood glucose to rise. Keep taking your diabetes medication and monitor your blood glucose frequently so that you know if you need to adjust your medication dosage or timing.

POSSIBLE CAUSES AND PREVENTION

A wide variety of factors may lead to hyperglycaemia. You can identify the specific cause of hyperglycaemic episodes that affect you by checking your blood glucose level regularly and relating the level to your circumstances at the time, which can help you prevent further episodes in the future.

CAUSE	PREVENTION

Food intake/ physical activity

Probably the most common causes of hyperglycaemia are an increase in the amount you eat (especially carbohydrates) or a decrease in physical activity, or a combination of both. Occasionally, an increase in physical activity may cause hyperglycaemia (see pp.104–105).

You can help to prevent hyperglycaemia by following healthy eating guidelines (see pp.74–75), staying active (see pp.100–103), and paying attention to balancing your food intake and medication. If you have type 2 diabetes that you manage with food and activity but find that your blood glucose is raised frequently, you should talk with your health professional because you may need to start taking medication to manage your diabetes.

Illness

When you are ill, more glucose is released by the liver into your bloodstream. Increased amounts of the stress hormones cortisol and adrenaline are also produced, which can interfere with the action of insulin, also causing your blood glucose to rise.

Frequent blood glucose monitoring when you are ill enables you to quickly adjust your diabetes treatment to compensate for your raised blood glucose level (see pp.70–71), or get advice from your health professional.

Stress/ hormonal changes

Stress hormones can disrupt the action of insulin, causing your blood glucose to rise. When you are stressed, you may also overeat or eat less healthy foods, which can also cause your blood glucose to rise. If you are a woman, you may find that your blood glucose rises at certain stages of your menstrual cycle (particularly just before periods). Hormonal changes during the menopause can also cause hyperglycaemia, as can some hormonal disorders, such as Cushing's syndrome (abnormally high levels of corticosteroid hormones).

If you find that stress or other hormonal changes raise your blood glucose, increase the frequency of blood glucose monitoring (or start monitoring, if you do not already do so) and, if your blood glucose is raised, take action by adjusting your diabetes treatment (see pp.70–71). If your hyperglycaemic episodes are due to hormonal changes, it may be possible to reduce the episodes by treating the underlying hormonal condition. Your health professional can help with this.

Diabetes medication

If you have not taken your insulin or other medication, your blood glucose rises. Sometimes, it may rise even if you have taken your insulin or medication correctly but it is no longer working effectively.

Ensuring you take your insulin or other medication as recommended is crucial to avoiding hyperglycaemia. If you have been doing this but still experience frequent hyperglycaemic episodes, your health professional may talk with you about, or advise changing to, a different dose or type of insulin or medication.

Hyperglycaemia is commonly caused by an increase in carbohydrate foods or a decrease in physical activity, or a combination of both

Recognizing and treating hyperglycaemia

High blood glucose – hyperglycaemia – is a characteristic feature of undiagnosed or under-treated diabetes. It is important to be able to identify and manage it promptly to bring your blood glucose down into your target range and so limit its short- and long-term effects.

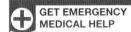
GET EMERGENCY MEDICAL HELP

- **Type 1 diabetes:** if your blood glucose is raised, you have symptoms of hyperglycaemia, and you have any level of ketones or cannot check for ketones.

- **Type 2 diabetes:** if your blood glucose is raised and/or you have symptoms of severe hyperglycaemia.

Symptoms of hyperglycaemia

The typical symptoms of hyperglycaemia are the same as those you may have had when diabetes was first diagnosed. However, hyperglycaemia does not always produce symptoms, especially if you have type 2 diabetes or your body has become accustomed to a raised blood glucose level.

Treating hyperglycaemia

If you develop hyperglycaemia, you need to tailor your treatment to its cause. This could mean eating less, increasing your level of physical activity, and/or increasing your dosage of insulin or other medication (see pp.48–51 for information about adjusting your insulin dose).

If you have type 2 diabetes that you manage through eating and physical activity, talk to your health professional if your blood glucose is consistently above 9 millimoles per litre (mmol/L) because you may need to start taking medication. If you are ill, treating your illness promptly should limit the effect of hyperglycaemia (see pp.124–125).

However you treat hyperglycaemia, checking your blood glucose frequently will tell you if it is returning to within its recommended range. If your blood glucose falls due to increasing your dosage of insulin or other medication, you may need to reduce the dosage when your blood glucose has returned to the recommended range. If you cannot discover the cause of your hyperglycaemia or are unsure about how to treat it, talk with your health professional.

Possible risks of hyperglycaemia

Brief episodes of hyperglycaemia are unlikely to be harmful, but a consistently high or rising blood glucose level (often due to illness, see pp.124–125) may

POSSIBLE SYMPTOMS OF HYPERGLYCAEMIA

Blurred vision

Frequently passing large amounts of urine

Tiredness and lack of energy

Recurrent infections or illnesses

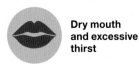
Dry mouth and excessive thirst

Weight loss

produce uncomfortable symptoms and may lead to diabetic ketoacidosis (DKA) if you have type 1 diabetes or hyperosmolar hyperglycaemic state (HHS) if you have type 2 diabetes. Both of these conditions need emergency medical treatment. In the long-term, a persistently raised blood glucose level increases your risk of developing diabetes-related complications (see pp.180–201).

Diabetic ketoacidosis (DKA)

If you have type 1 diabetes and there is no insulin in your body, your body cells cannot take in glucose and break down fat as an alternative source of energy. During this breakdown, toxic by-products called ketones are produced, which, in addition to extreme thirst and frequent passing of urine, can cause unpleasant symptoms, including:
• Nausea and vomiting.
• Abdominal pain.
• Fruity-smelling breath and impaired consciousness in the later stages.
Without prompt medical treatment, DKA can lead to a life-threatening coma.

If you have any symptoms of DKA, check your blood glucose level. If it is above 11 mmol/L, you should also check your ketone level if you have the appropriate equipment.

Hyperosmolar hyperglycaemic state (HHS)

If you have type 2 diabetes, you are less likely to develop DKA because you may still produce some insulin. The presence of some insulin means that your body cells still have access to glucose and do not need to break down fat for energy, so they do not produce ketones. However, severe hyperglycaemia can

CHECKING KETONES

You can check for ketones either in your urine or your blood. Urine testing requires strips that you dip into a urine sample; the strip changes colour, and the colour is compared against a chart to give a ketone reading. Blood ketones are checked in the same way as blood glucose, using a fingerprick blood sample, test strips, and a meter. Some blood glucose meters are also able to measure ketones; alternatively, a dedicated ketone meter may be used.

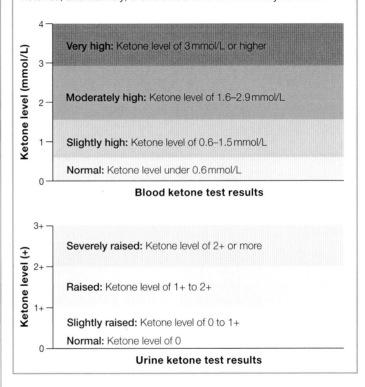

Blood ketone test results

Very high: Ketone level of 3 mmol/L or higher

Moderately high: Ketone level of 1.6–2.9 mmol/L

Slightly high: Ketone level of 0.6–1.5 mmol/L

Normal: Ketone level under 0.6 mmol/L

Urine ketone test results

Severely raised: Ketone level of 2+ or more

Raised: Ketone level of 1+ to 2+

Slightly raised: Ketone level of 0 to 1+

Normal: Ketone level of 0

lead to a serious condition known as hyperosmolar hyperglycaemic state (HHS), with symptoms that may include:
• Dehydration and dry skin.
• Thirst.
• Frequent passing of urine.
• Nausea.
• Confusion and disorientation; if severe, HHS may cause loss of consciousness.
Without prompt medical treatment, HHS can lead to extreme dehydration and coma, and can be life-threatening.

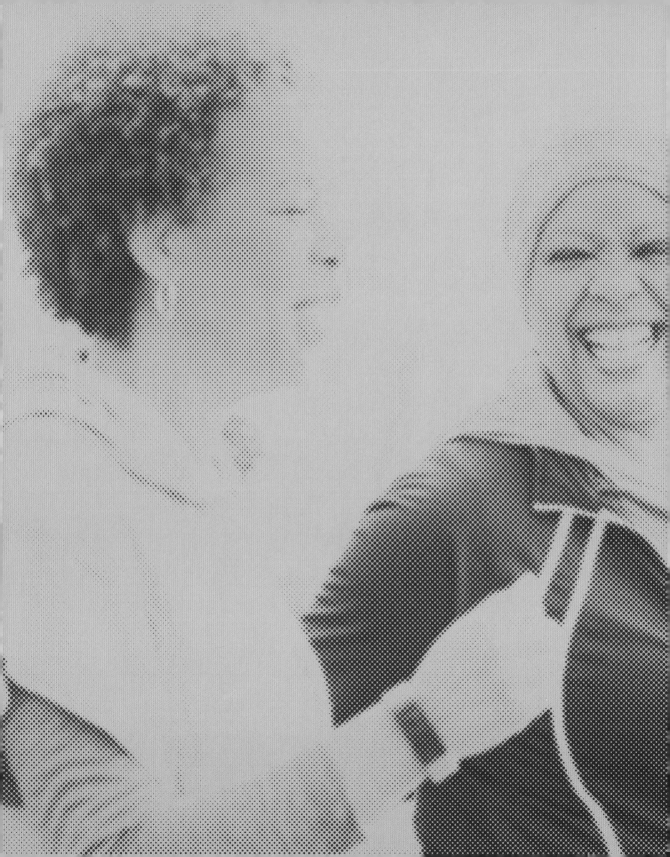

Eating, drinking, and being active

Healthy eating

The basic principles of healthy eating if you have diabetes are no different to those for anyone else. However, it's good to be familiar with the main food groups and how to balance your food intake to be as healthy as possible. Eating healthily is one of the key factors in reducing the risk of heart disease and other complications.

The importance of healthy eating

There are some basic principles underlying good nutrition and a healthy diet, and these are helpful to follow no matter what type of diabetes you have. Understanding food groups (see panel, opposite) is useful and more information about these groups is given on the following pages.

By following some general healthy eating tips (see below), you can quickly adopt good habits that will help keep your cholesterol and blood glucose levels within a healthy range and help to reduce the risk of diabetes complications.

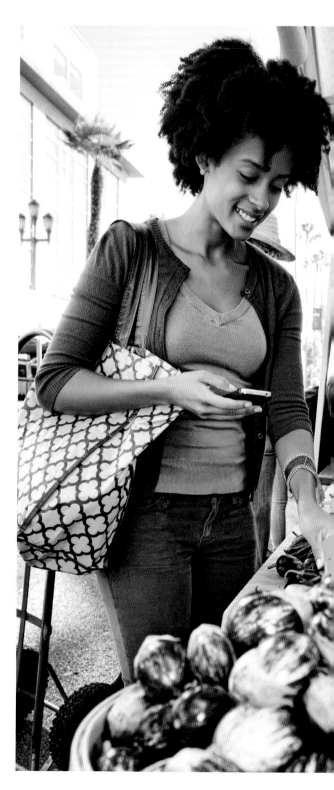

HEALTHY EATING TIPS

- Limit the amount of table sugar and sugary foods you consume.

- Watch out for hidden carbohydrates, especially in fruit drinks.

- Eat regular meals that contain some complex carbohydrate.

- Choose healthier carbohydrates such as brown rice, chickpeas, lentils, and vegetables.

- Cut down on fat, especially saturated fats.

- Eat more high-fibre foods, including fruit and vegetables.

- Try to have homemade meals rather than ready-made meals several times a week.

- Reduce red meat in your everyday eating.

- Reduce your salt intake to help prevent high blood pressure.

- Keep your alcohol consumption within the recommended limits.

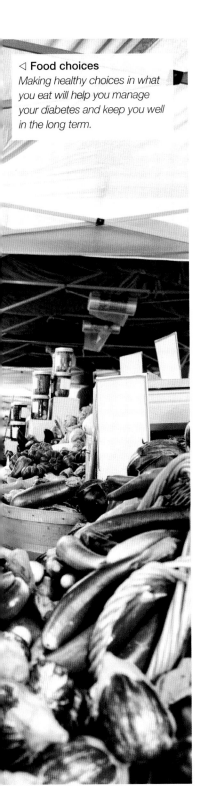

◁ Food choices
Making healthy choices in what you eat will help you manage your diabetes and keep you well in the long term.

A balanced diet

You can achieve a balanced diet by eating a variety of foods from each of the main food groups: proteins, carbohydrates, and fats. There are no strict recommendations about the proportion of each, but there are general guidelines. In the UK*, these state that starchy carbohydrates (such as grains, cereals, potatoes, and bread) and fruit and vegetables should make up the bulk of meals – about two-thirds of a plate. Protein-rich foods, such as eggs, pulses, fish, or lean meat, should form a smaller part of each meal. You should aim to have at least five portions of fruit and vegetables a day (one portion being 80 g) – an apple, a handful of berries, or three tablespoons of peas, for example. Fruit and vegetables are low in calories and rich in vitamins and minerals, although fruit does contain some natural sugar. Sugar, salt, and saturated fat are ideally eaten only in small amounts.

FOOD GROUPS

There are three main food groups – carbohydrates (simple and complex), fats, and protein. Individual foods may contain more than one of these food types, although one component usually predominates.

CATEGORY	ROLE AND MAIN SOURCES
Carbohydrate	Carbohydrates are used by the body for energy. They fall into two types: simple and complex. Complex carbohydrates take longer to digest and help you feel full. Simple carbohydrates include table sugar and honey. Complex carbohydrates include grains, cereals, and many vegetables. See also pp.78–83.
Fat	Fat is an important component of many body cells and plays a key role in growth and development. There are different types: saturated and unsaturated. Unsaturated fat is healthiest. Fat is found in oils, butter, and spreads, as well as in red meat, fish, dairy produce and eggs, and in nuts and seeds. See also p.84.
Protein	Your body needs protein to create, maintain, and repair its cells. The main sources of protein are meat, fish, beans and other pulses, nuts, eggs, and dairy products. See also p.85.

Food and diabetes

Learning about how some foods can affect your diabetes and developing a knowledge of what meals and snacks work best for you are key when you have diabetes. If you take insulin or insulin-stimulating tablets, you need to be aware of how food interacts with insulin. If you are overweight, then paying attention to your food intake is important if you are trying to lose weight.

Type 1 diabetes

If you have type 1 diabetes, matching your food intake to the action of your insulin is the way to maintain a healthy blood glucose level. For example, if you take a shorter-acting insulin, you will need to take it around the time that you are having your meals. You will also be taking a longer-acting insulin, and you may need to eat extra snacks to make sure that there is glucose available in your body when your insulin is working at its peak. The exact timing of your food and insulin together will depend on the type of insulin you take (see pp.44–45).

> **PLANNING FOOD INTAKE**
>
> Set aside some time each week to plan your food intake.
>
> - If you think you won't be able to get something to eat when your tablets or insulin are working, take food with you from home.
> - Balance your food intake through the day rather than having one very large meal, which could cause your blood glucose level to rise too high.
> - If you choose a sugary snack, eat it with or after other types of food (such as after a main course) to reduce its impact on your blood glucose level.

Type 2 diabetes

With type 2 diabetes, your body's ability to produce insulin effectively when you eat is impaired, so eating foods that take longer to be broken down into glucose can help your pancreas to cope. Sugary foods are converted into glucose fastest so eating them after a meal, when your body is already slowly digesting other food, can help to reduce their impact on blood glucose. Avoiding eating a lot of carbohydrate-rich food at once helps to reduce the pressure on your pancreas.

If you are taking tablets for your diabetes, you will need to take them in relation to your meals, because some work by helping your body to break down food more slowly, whereas others make your pancreas produce more insulin (see p.59). If you are taking insulin for your type 2 diabetes, you need to be aware of its peak of action (see p.45) so you can time eating to prevent a hypo.

If you are overweight, you may also need to change your food intake in order to lose weight (see pp.94–99).

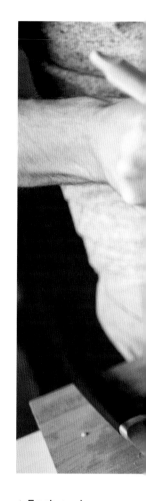

△ **Fresh produce**
Making your own meals with lots of fresh produce gives you more control over what you eat. Salads are a great way to fill up. Get inspiration for recipes from books or online resources.

If your eating habit is irregular or disrupted, your blood glucose level may also be erratic

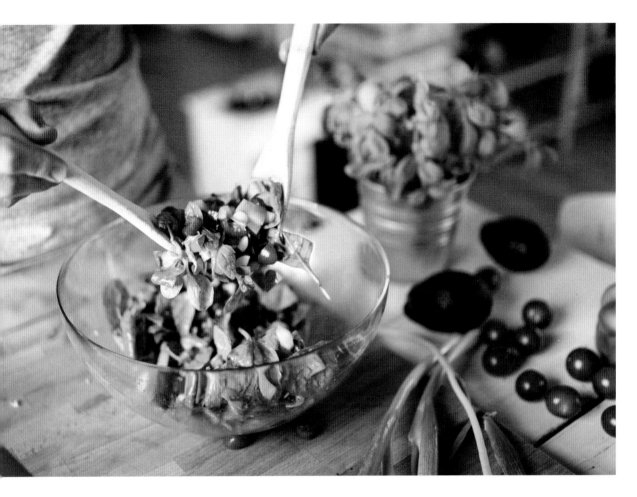

Timing of meals and snacking

An important part of living with diabetes is recognizing when you need to eat or drink in order to balance the effects of tablets or insulin on your blood glucose. Regularly eating meals that contain complex carbohydrate will fuel your body, help your digestive system to function properly, and avoid sharp changes in your blood glucose level.

Having diabetes doesn't mean you eat more snacks, but they may be necessary if you use insulin or insulin-stimulating tablets and you need to avoid becoming hypoglycaemic. Try to make sure that snacks aren't high in fat or sugar.

SNACKS UNDER 100 CALORIES

 20 grapes

 20g salted or plain popcorn

 160g mango

 1 large apple

 20g dried fruit and nuts

 2 small oranges

 4 bread sticks

 1 medium banana

Carbohydrates and fibre

Carbohydrates are an essential energy source for the body, but they can have a significant effect on blood glucose levels. Fibre can also affect blood glucose levels, because it has an impact on how quickly carbohydrates are absorbed.

Types of carbohydrate

Carbohydrates fall into two categories: simple carbohydrates, also known as sugars, and complex carbohydrates, also known as starches. Simple carbohydrates are digested and absorbed into the blood rapidly, whereas complex carbohydrates are digested and absorbed more slowly.

Simple carbohydrates

The main simple carbohydrates are the sugars glucose, sucrose, fructose, and lactose. Because they are broken down and absorbed quickly, they can cause your blood glucose level to rise sharply, creating an immediate demand for more insulin. However, this effect is useful if you need to treat a hypo (see pp.66–67).

Sugar is in many products, such as sweets, chocolate, non-diet soft drinks, and cakes. "Natural" forms occur in honey, fruit, and milk. Many processed foods – even savoury ones – also contain sugars. Eating sugary foods with or after other food will slow their absorption. Choosing foods with less sugar (see Checking food labels, p.96) will help to prevent blood glucose spikes.

Carbohydrates have a major effect on blood glucose levels

Complex carbohydrates

These are found in foods such as rice, pasta, wholegrain bread, potatoes, cereals, beans, and pulses. Like simple carbohydrates, they are also broken down into glucose but they are digested more slowly and so do not cause a spike in blood glucose. However, refined (processed) carbohydrates – found in white bread, cakes, and most pastries, for example – have had the bran and kernel of the grain removed, leaving just the starch. These are digested faster than unprocessed grains, and they may raise blood glucose levels almost as quickly as simple sugars.

ARTIFICIAL SWEETENERS

You can use artificial sweeteners instead of sugar to sweeten food and drinks such as tea and coffee. These products contain aspartame, saccharin, cyclamate, acesulfame K, or sucralose, none of which affect your blood glucose. These products are classed as food additives and have been tested for safety. Because of this, each type of sweetener has a recommended daily amount (shown on the label) that should not be exceeded. If you use sweeteners instead of sugar in recipes, bear in mind that they lose their sweetness if heated to high temperatures so are best added after cooking.

SIMPLE CARBOHYDRATES (SUGARS)

These are rapidly absorbed and cause a sharp rise in blood glucose levels, but are useful to treat a hypo caused by too much insulin. Many processed foods contain hidden sugars.

 Sugar: all types, including palm, muscovado, and brown sugar.

 Honey and syrups, including corn syrup, and agave nectar.

 Jams: most contain more than 60% sugar; some low-sugar jams may contain less than 10% sugar.

 Sweets and chocolate have varying, but generally large, amounts of added sugar.

 Sugary drinks, including squash and fizzy drinks, contain high levels of sugar.

 Cakes, biscuits, and desserts often contain a high proportion of sugar.

 Fruits contain the fruit sugar fructose. Berries have low levels, while pineapple, mango, and melon are high in fructose.

 Milk and yoghurt: cows' milk (all types, unflavoured) contains 5% lactose; yoghurts may be sweetened with sugar or fruit purée.

 Fruit juice contains fruit sugar (fructose), which is rapidly absorbed.

COMPLEX CARBOHYDRATES (STARCHES)

These are broken down in the digestive system into glucose, but unprocessed forms are digested relatively slowly so do not cause a dramatic rise in blood glucose.

 Bread (including naan, pitta, and chappatis): wholegrain varieties are digested more slowly than refined types.

 Rice: brown and wild rice are broken down more slowly than white rice.

 Pasta and couscous are both wheat-based products. Wholewheat pasta is broken down more slowly than ordinary pasta.

 Noodles: wheat and egg noodles are usually made from refined carbohydrates.

 Potatoes, plantains, and yams contain natural forms of complex carbohydrate.

 Oats: eaten as porridge or used in other products, oats are also high in soluble fibre (see p.83).

 Beans (including haricot, borlotti, and kidney beans) contain fibre as well as carbohydrate. This slows digestion.

 Lentils: these are good sources of protein as well as carbohydrate.

 Bulgur wheat and quinoa: bulgur (a wholegrain cereal) and quinoa (a nutrient-rich seed eaten like a grain) are digested slowly.

Managing your carbohydrate intake

Carbohydrates have a significant impact on your blood glucose level, so you need to be aware of the carbohydrate content of what you eat. Being aware of your intake can help you in managing your diabetes, whatever type it is. Monitoring and limiting your carbohydrate intake can be a good way to lose weight if you need to, or to prevent or delay type 2 diabetes. Foods with no carbohydrate do not tend to affect blood glucose levels.

Carbohydrate counting (see p.82) is an important method for matching the amount of insulin you need to take. While carbohydrate content will have the most effect on your blood glucose, considering the glycaemic index (GI) of food can also be useful – for example, if you are having unexpected swings of blood glucose.

Low GI foods are not always a healthy choice. Peanuts, for example, are high in fat.

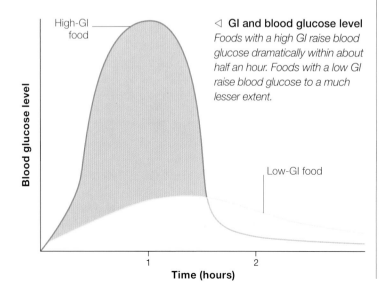

◁ **GI and blood glucose level**
Foods with a high GI raise blood glucose dramatically within about half an hour. Foods with a low GI raise blood glucose to a much lesser extent.

High-GI food

Low-GI food

Blood glucose level

1 2
Time (hours)

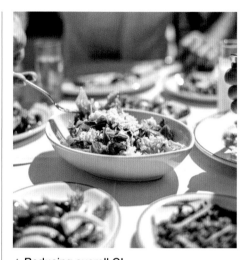

△ **Reducing overall GI**
The GI applies to a specific food eaten on its own. Eating a low GI food together with a high one can reduce the overall GI.

Understanding glycaemic index (GI)

The GI is a ranking of carbohydrate-containing foods based on their effect on blood glucose level. Foods that are digested slowly have a low GI rating; quickly digested foods have a high rating (see chart opposite). Eating more low- and medium-GI foods can help you balance your blood glucose level.

Higher-GI foods tend to be those that are higher in refined sugar. These foods can cause spikes in your blood glucose level. On the other hand, not all lower-GI foods are healthy options. For example, a flapjack is made with low-GI oats, but also contains a lot of sugar and fat; chocolate has a low GI because the fat slows its absorption.

The GI applies to an individual food; when foods of differing GIs are mixed, high-GI foods are absorbed more slowly than when eaten on their own. Cooking methods and ripeness can also affect the GI of a food.

GLYCAEMIC INDEX

Foods are given a GI number between 1 and 100, with glucose (sugar) scoring 100 because it causes blood glucose to rise very quickly.

Each food has a GI rating, and different brands of the same food can vary. The following foods are examples of each category.

HIGHER-GI FOODS (OVER 70)

Mashed potatoes

Honey

Popcorn

Potato crisps

Watermelons

Noodles

Full-sugar cola

MEDIUM-GI FOODS (55–69)

Raisins

Brown bread

Boiled potatoes (with skin)

Melons

Bananas

Couscous

White rice

LOWER-GI FOODS (UNDER 55)

White pasta

Sweet potatoes

Brown rice

Basmati rice

Rye bread

Peas

Kidney beans

Yoghurt

Dried apricots

Chickpeas

Lentils

Dark chocolate (70% cocoa)

Red peppers

Onions

Aubergines

MAKING GI WORK FOR YOU

- When planning meals, work out whether most of the meal is higher GI or lower GI, so that you can predict its effect on your blood glucose.

- Remember that if you eat only very low-GI foods you may need to reduce your insulin or medication dose in order to avoid unexpected hypos.

- Experiment with different foods to find their GI effect, by checking your blood glucose after eating them.

- Eating a higher-GI food together with or after lower-GI one (for example, a sweet dessert after a complex carbohydrate) can reduce the effect of the higher-GI food on your blood glucose level.

Carbohydrate counting

You can use carbohydrate counting to help you calculate how much insulin you need to take to cover a meal. This will help you to prevent a blood glucose spike. This technique is especially important if you are using rapid-acting insulins and gives you more freedom about what you eat. First, identify the foods that don't contain carbohydrate (for example, lean meat, butter, and cheese) as they don't need to be counted. Then work out the total carbohydrate content of each of the individual carbohydrate-containing foods. Finally, use your personal insulin:carbohydrate ratio (see p.49) to calculate your insulin dose. For example, if you need 1 unit of insulin per 10g carbohydrate, you will need 4.5 units for a meal that has 45g of carbohydrate.

Carbohydrate-counting tools

Various tools are available to help you count your carbohydrate intake. You can refer to carbohydrate reference tables (available as booklets and online) or food labels (see p.96). There are also apps that can calculate the amount of carbohydrate for you.

HOW TO COUNT CARBOHYDRATES

By adding up the carbohydrate in each food, you can find the total amount for each meal. This will enable you to calculate how much bolus insulin you need, using your insulin:carbohydrate ratio.

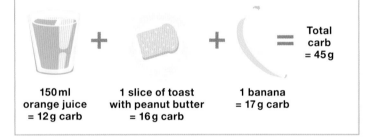

| 150 ml orange juice = 12 g carb | 1 slice of toast with peanut butter = 16 g carb | 1 banana = 17 g carb | Total carb = 45 g |

UNDERSTANDING CARBOHYDRATE CONTENT

The more carbohydrate your food contains, the more insulin you need to convert it into energy. Carbohydrate content always stays the same, regardless of how it is cooked – although the food will weigh more if it absorbs water during cooking. Always try to count the carbohydrate content of raw food rather than cooked.

AMOUNT	EXAMPLES OF FOODS
10 g carbohydrate	1 thin slice bread; 1 crispbread; 3 small pretzels; 1 digestive biscuit; 18g popcorn; 16g tortilla chips; 1 taco shell; 1 tablespoon rice (uncooked); 30g tagliatelle (uncooked); 2 tablespoons beans; 1 small apple; 1 level scoop ice-cream.
15 g carbohydrate	1 medium slice bread; 1 boiled potato (90g); 1 crumpet or muffin; 1 mini chocolate muffin; 19g marshmallow; 2 x 25g poppadoms; 95g spaghetti (uncooked); 1 medium grapefruit; 1 banana (73g) ; 284ml milk.
20 g carbohydrate	1 thick slice bread; 1 large croissant; 1 mini pitta; 60g pasta twists (uncooked); 70g rice noodles (uncooked); 100g quiche Lorraine; 1 mango; 2 tablespoons raisins; 4 jelly babies or jelly beans.
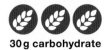 **30 g carbohydrate**	1 bagel; 1 large scone; 1 wholemeal tortilla; 1 mini naan; 92g gnocchi; 1 cup bran cereal; 2 tablespoons lentils (uncooked); 100 g oven chips; 4 slices pineapple; 8–10 dried apricots; 30 grapes; 48g dark chocolate.

Fibre

There are two types of dietary fibre, both of which are important to your health. Insoluble fibre helps food to pass through your digestive system, thus keeping your intestines healthy and reducing the risk of constipation. Soluble fibre slows the digestion of carbohydrate and stops your blood glucose level from rising too quickly after eating. Soluble fibre also helps to reduce your cholesterol level. Many fibre-rich foods contain both types of fibre, but one type tends to dominate.

Adults should aim to eat around 30 g of fibre a day. If you need to increase your fibre intake, do so gradually, and drink plenty of fluids with the food.

Fruit and vegetables

As well as being low in calories and rich in vitamins and minerals, fruit and vegetables are excellent sources of fibre.

Including the skin of fruit and vegetables – such as apple peel and potato skins – will help to increase your fibre intake. Space out your consumption of fruit and vegetables through the day to get the nutritional benefits without raising your blood glucose level too much.

HOW TO ADD MORE FIBRE TO YOUR DIET

- Add extra fruit, seeds, or nuts to breakfast cereals and yoghurts.
- Add beans or lentils to dishes such as stews and curries. This will also reduce the meat and fat content of these meals.
- Include plenty of vegetables with meals.
- Keep chopped raw vegetables, such as carrots, celery, and cherry tomatoes, prepared in the refrigerator for snacks.
- Choose unprocessed grains, such as wholegrain pasta and rice.

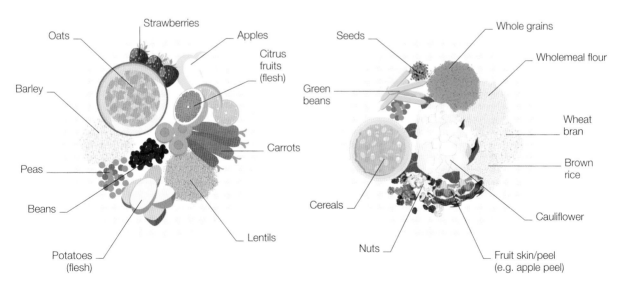

△ **Good sources of soluble fibre**
Many foods that are high in soluble fibre are useful as snacks on their own or can be added to mealtime dishes to make them healthier and stretch further.

△ **Good sources of insoluble fibre**
Foods that are high in insoluble fibre tend to increase the feeling of fullness, so can help to prevent you from feeling hungry between meals. They can also help to prevent constipation.

Fats, proteins, vitamins, and minerals

Fats and proteins are important components of any eating plan. Although they don't have a direct effect on blood sugar, fats are high in calories. Understanding which protein foods are healthiest and trying to avoid the most unhealthy fats is important for anyone with diabetes.

HOW TO CUT DOWN ON FAT

- Replace butter or full-fat margarines with lower-fat spreads, particularly products that contain monounsaturated fats.

- Use low-fat crème fraîche, Greek yoghurt, or low-fat fromage frais.

- Eat more fish, including two portions of oily fish a week.

- Choose lean cuts of meat and skinless poultry.

- Avoid eating fried foods.

Fat in your diet

Fats are found in dairy products, such as milk, butter, and cheese, cooking oils, meats, and nuts, as well as in processed foods. Fats have little effect on blood glucose but there are good reasons to limit your fat intake when you have diabetes. Eating too much fat is linked to high blood levels of fat (hyperlipidaemia), heart and circulatory disease, and stroke, all of which are possible complications of diabetes (see pp.192–197). Being overweight can also contribute to the risk of developing these complications, and fats are very high in calories. While dairy products are high in fat, they also contain carbohydrate and protein and are a source of calcium and vitamins.

To help protect against heart and circulatory conditions, and also to help if you are trying to lose weight, choose lower-fat versions of fatty foods, for example, semi-skimmed milk, low-fat or fat-free yoghurt, or reduced-fat cheese.

TYPES OF FATS

HEALTHIER FATS

Monounsaturated fats

Monounsaturated fats are found in some margarines and cooking oils, including olive oil and rapeseed (canola) oil. They are also in nuts, seeds, and avocados. These fats do not raise levels of LDL ("bad") cholesterol and are a healthier alternative to saturated fats.

Polyunsaturated fats

There are two groups of polyunsaturated fatty acids: omega-3 and omega-6. Omega-3 is found in oily fish, rapeseed oil, and walnuts. Omega-6 is found in sunflower, safflower, and corn oils. They are healthier than saturated fats.

LESS HEALTHY FATS

Saturated fats

Saturated fats are mainly found in animal products – butter, cheese, and the fat around a piece of steak are examples – but they are also found in coconut and palm oils. These fats raise blood levels of LDL ("bad") cholesterol.

Trans fats

Often listed on food labels as partially hydrogenated or hydrogenated fat, trans fats are found in many processed foods, such as biscuits and cakes, and in deep-fried food. They raise LDL ("bad") cholesterol levels, and eating many foods that are high in trans fats is linked to an increased risk of a heart attack.

Proteins

Protein is a vital nutrient: your body needs it to create, maintain, and repair its cells, and to keep your muscles healthy. To eat healthily, you need about 1 g of protein per kilogram of your body weight – for example, if you weigh 80 kg, you need 80 g protein per day. Protein has little effect on your blood glucose level, but when you are choosing which type to eat, you can make healthier choices – for example, by cutting down on red meat,

Fruit and vegetables are excellent sources of vitamins and minerals. Many are also high in antioxidants, which may help to counteract insulin resistance. They may also help to protect against circulatory conditions, although this has not been scientifically proven.

▽ **Protein sources**
The main sources of protein in food are meat, fish, eggs and dairy produce, and beans and other pulses. Some of these are high in fat so should be eaten in only limited amounts.

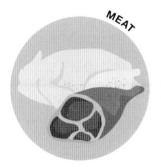

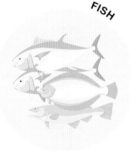

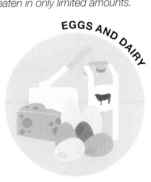

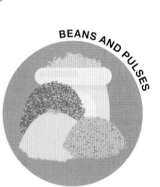

Although high in protein, some meat is high in fat. Poultry is a low-fat choice.

Fish are a low-fat protein source. Oily fish contain omega-3 fatty acids.

Eggs, cheese, and milk are good protein sources but also contain fats.

Beans and other pulses are low in fat and high in fibre as well as protein.

eating reduced-fat cheese, and including oily fish in your meals two to three times a week. Milk, cheese, and yoghurt also have lots of calcium as well as protein. If you enjoy eggs, have them scrambled (without using butter), poached, or boiled to avoid consuming extra fat.

Vitamins and minerals

A healthy, balanced food intake provides all the vitamins and minerals you need. Whether you have diabetes or not, you do not need to take vitamin or mineral supplements unless your registered health professional advises it. Supplements may be recommended if your food intake is restricted in any way.

SALT

Having diabetes increases your risk of developing high blood pressure and other circulatory conditions, and eating too much salt also increases this risk. If you have been diagnosed with high blood pressure, you will be asked to reduce your salt intake. Using less or no salt in cooking, and not adding salt at the table, will help you keep your salt intake within the recommended daily amount of no more than 6 g (the equivalent of one teaspoon). Hidden sources of salt include processed foods, and ready meals often have especially high amounts.

Drinks

As well as the food you eat each day, some drinks can affect your blood glucose and you may need to keep track of how much of these you consume. Many sweet, fizzy drinks and alcoholic drinks are high in sugar and calories.

Non-alcoholic drinks

You can safely drink tea, herbal tea, black coffee, and water without affecting your diabetes. These will help keep you hydrated. By limiting the amount of milk you take in teas and coffees, and drinking them with skimmed or semi-skimmed milk, you will cut down on calories. If you don't like water, you can try adding lemon or mint to it, to add some flavour, or drink herbal tea.

Some drinks have hidden calories and sugar, so try to keep these to a minimum. Sugary, fizzy drinks are high in sugar; switching to sugar-free or low-sugar varieties will help. Fruit juices and smoothies contain natural fruit sugars, which also affect your blood glucose level – juices can easily be diluted. Sugar-free squash and cordials are useful substitutes for pure fruit juice and don't affect your blood glucose.

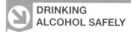

DRINKING ALCOHOL SAFELY

Take the following steps to help reduce the impact of alcohol:

- Eat a carbohydrate-containing meal before you start drinking.
- If you can't eat before you have a drink, make sure you have snacks that contain carbohydrate, such as sandwiches or crisps, while you are drinking.
- Carry glucose with you in case you have a hypo. Having diabetes ID is also useful.
- If you're driving, don't drink any alcohol at all.
- If you drink more than a few units of alcohol in the evening, always have a snack before going to sleep.

GET EMERGENCY MEDICAL HELP

- Drinking too much alcohol can cause a hypo, which may be mistaken for drunkenness and can be severe. If a person has been drinking alcohol and you think they are having a hypo, call for emergency medical help.

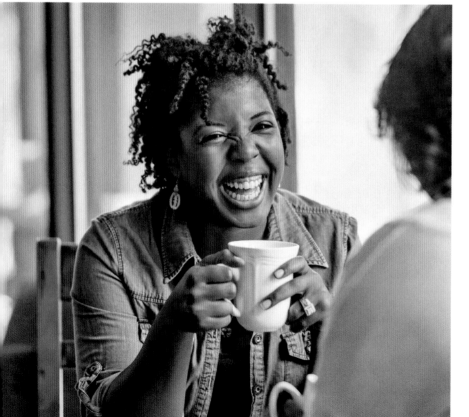

◁ **Socializing with a drink**
Keep track of what you drink when you go out. High-sugar drinks or adding sugar to drinks can cause a spike in your blood glucose levels.

Alcohol

There's no reason why you shouldn't drink alcohol when you have diabetes. However, you need to be aware of its potential impact (see below), and drink within recommended limits. This means having no more than 14 units of alcohol spread out over a week, with some alcohol-free days each week.

Alcohol raises your blood glucose level initially, but in larger quantities it prevents your liver from releasing glucose from its stores, lowering blood glucose and making a hypo last longer and be more severe; this may be serious and happen while you're asleep. You can reduce the risk of a hypo by eating a carbohydrate-containing meal before or while you are drinking, or having snacks, particularly if you drink more than 1–3 units of alcohol. You may need to take a smaller dose of insulin or insulin-stimulating tablets if you think you might be drinking more than 3 units. It is better to have a slightly higher blood glucose level for a short time than suffer a serious hypo that might need hospital treatment.

TYPES OF ALCOHOLIC DRINK AND EFFECT ON BLOOD GLUCOSE

Alcohol contains simple carbohydrate (sugar), so drinking will initially raise your blood glucose level – the higher the alcohol content, the greater the effect. Many alcoholic drinks are high in calories and carbohydrate content. The alcohol percentage varies, so check the alcohol content given on labels of beers and wines.

DRINK	CALS	CARBOHYDRATE	ALCOHOL CONTENT AND UNITS	EFFECT ON BLOOD GLUCOSE
Beer (1 pint)	140–185	9–14g	4.5% (2 units)	Causes an initial rise in your blood glucose level. Ordinary bitter has less effect on your blood glucose than strong or real ale.
Lager (1 pint)	170–230	7.5g	3.2–4% (2 units)	Causes an initial rise in your blood glucose level. Low-carb/diet lagers will not raise your blood glucose but can be high in alcohol.
Dry white wine (small glass, 125ml)	80–90	0.7g	9–14.5% (1–1.5 units)	Dry and sweet wines contain similar amounts of alcohol but dry wine has less effect on your blood glucose level because it contains less sugar.
Sweet white wine (small glass, 125ml)	110–120	7.5g	9–14.5% (1–1.5 units)	
Red wine (small glass, 125ml)	110–120	0.4g	9–14.5% (1–1.5 units)	Red wine contains less carbohydrate than white wine but the effect on your blood glucose level is similar.
Spirits (single measure, 25ml)	50	Trace	40–60% (1 unit)	All spirits have similar amounts of alcohol and calories. On their own, they do not greatly raise your blood glucose level.
Dry sherry (25ml)	58	Trace	15.5–20% (1 unit)	Dry sherries have less effect on your blood glucose than sweet varieties.
Sweet sherry (25ml)	68	3.5g	15.5–20% (1 unit)	

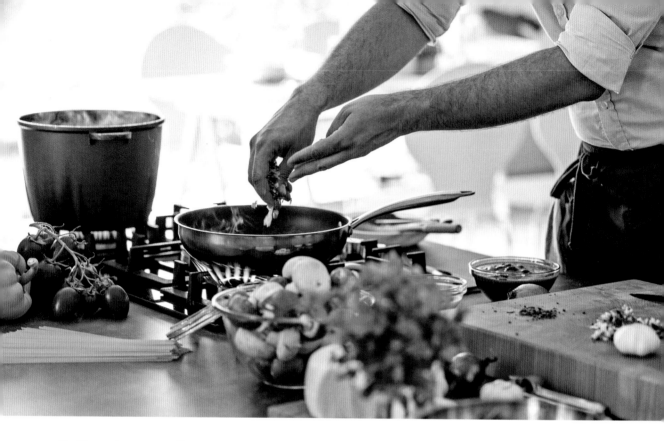

Cooking and eating out

Having diabetes doesn't mean that you have to miss out on your favourite recipes. Instead, you can adapt them to reduce your fat, salt, and sugar consumption, and include more fruit and vegetables to make your meals healthy and well-balanced. Even for special events, such as a party, dining out, or a festive occasion, you can make choices that enable you to enjoy your food and still stay well.

Healthier cooking

To limit your fat intake, try to grill, steam, or bake foods rather than fry them. If a recipe does require frying, use cooking oil instead of butter (see p.84 for healthier types of fats). If roasting meat, place it on a rack to let the fat drain away. Adding herbs helps you to bring out the flavour in food, and use less salt. You don't have to leave out every high-fat or high-sugar food, however, especially if a little of that ingredient goes a long way. Parmesan cheese, for example, is high in fat but has a very strong flavour – you only need to use a sprinkling. Honey, too, is high in sugar, but a small amount can sweeten a dish more effectively than a lot of sugar. So if a recipe calls for small amounts of high-fat or high-sugar ingredients, go ahead and use them.

Festivals and celebrations

With planning, you can fit your diabetes care in to any celebratory event. First, find out the timings when food will be served; then you can work out (with help from your health professional if you need it) the timings of your insulin and/or tablets and monitoring to match. For example, for a late-afternoon wedding with a sit-down meal, you may need to take your evening medication a little later than usual, while for a lunchtime celebration, you may need extra blood glucose checks and to be prepared with your own snacks in case of delay in eating. You may also need an extra dose of tablets or insulin in advance, if you know you'll be eating a lot.

Some religious events involve fasting and then eating at set times. Although having diabetes can exempt you, if you still want to fast you can manage by having lower doses of your diabetes medication before fasting and changing the time for doses after the fast, while also monitoring your blood glucose regularly. Drink plenty of sugar-free fluids, including during the fast if possible, to avoid dehydration.

Dancing, drinking alcohol, or delays in eating can all make a hypo more likely (see pp.62–67). To prevent a hypo or to stop one from becoming more severe, it is important for you to carry hypo remedies and to be alert for any symptoms.

With planning, you can fit your diabetes care in to any celebratory event

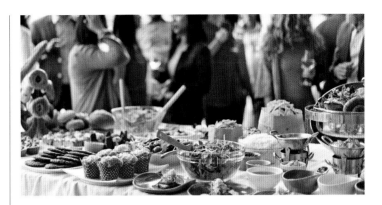

RECIPE ADJUSTMENTS

There are low-fat, low-sugar substitutes for many ingredients. There are also cooking methods that reduce calories without compromising flavour.

- Use more vegetables in soups and stews to increase fibre and reduce fat content. Instead of adding cream, add a little low-fat yoghurt at the end of cooking.

- Use half-fat crème fraîche instead of cream (for example, in home-made ice cream).

- Use strongly flavoured cheese in recipes, such as parmesan, goats' cheese, or feta, so that you don't need to use as much.

- If using a fatty meat, dry-fry it first and drain off the excess fat before continuing with the recipe.

- Use tomato-based sauces for pasta dishes rather than cream.

- If using pastry, just use a thin single layer (for example, with a pie) or use a potato topping for a savoury dish instead.

- Cut down the amount of salt you use; replace it with herbs, spices, or lemon juice to add flavour.

- Use virtually fat-free fromage frais and reduced-fat cream cheese in equal amounts instead of eggs and mascarpone cheese to make tiramisu. You can still add a small amount of sugar.

- Cut down the amount of sugar in pudding recipes or substitute artificial sweeteners (check the packet for when to add these).

△ **Festivities and food**
Celebrations often have lots of tempting foods you want to try. Plan in advance how to manage your diabetes so that your blood glucose stays in your target range, even if you eat more than usual.

Eating out

You don't need to deny yourself the pleasure of eating out, especially if you do so only occasionally. One way to allow for extra food and drink is to adjust your medication to allow for a rise in your blood glucose level if necessary. Even if you don't, the rise will be brief and your blood glucose level will lower again once you return to your usual eating pattern.

The timing of a meal out may differ from your normal mealtimes. This means you may need to change the time of your tablets or insulin injection to coordinate your dose with your food intake. You may not be able to predict exactly when you will be eating, but you can alter the usual timing by around two hours without it affecting your overall blood glucose level. If you delay your medication, however, it may continue working later than normal as a result. Take a snack with you or plan what to do in case the service is slow, to avoid having a hypo while you are waiting.

Choosing from the menu

If you are keen to keep to healthy eating, the following ideas may help:
- **Fats** Avoid dishes that are deep-fried or drenched in sauce or oil.
- **Meat** If possible, ask for extra vegetables and a little less meat.
- **Sauces** Order sauces in a separate jug so that you can control the amount.
- **Fruit and vegetables** Opt for fruit- or vegetable-based dishes, or ask for extra amounts.
- **Drinks** Have low-calorie drinks or water rather than, or together with, alcohol or fruit juice.

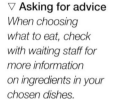
▽ **Asking for advice**
When choosing what to eat, check with waiting staff for more information on ingredients in your chosen dishes.

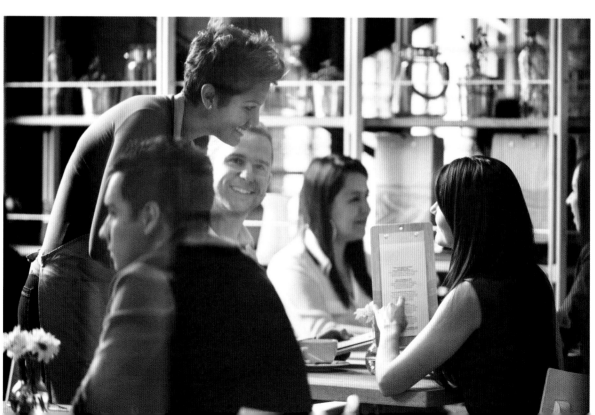

HEALTHY MENU OPTIONS

Every restaurant menu should have options that fit into a healthy-eating plan. On the whole, vegetable-based dishes are healthier than meat dishes, and fruit-based desserts are better than those with a lot of cream, sugar, or pastry. You also need to consider what foods accompany your dish, so that your meal is balanced. Ask the restaurant staff for advice if you need more information about portion size, ingredients, or cooking methods. It is especially important to bear healthy menu options in mind if you eat out regularly. The table below gives examples of healthy and less healthy choices for each type of dish.

HEALTHY CHOICES		LESS HEALTHY CHOICES
 Meat dishes	Steak without sauce; roast chicken (skin removed); grilled lamb (fat removed); stir-fried pork with vegetables; kebabs (no sauce); tikka or tandoori meats.	Beef stroganoff; steak and kidney pie; steak in creamy sauce; fried lamb chops; burger in a bun; curries with creamy sauces (such as korma).
 Fish dishes	Baked or poached salmon or tuna; grilled swordfish steak; smoked mackerel fillets; tuna salad; potato-topped fish pie; sashimi or sushi rolls with no rice.	Fish in batter; deep-fried scampi; fish in creamy sauce; fish in cheese-based sauce; "California roll" sushi pieces; tempura dishes.
 Pasta and noodle dishes	Pasta with vegetable or tomato sauce; spaghetti Bolognese; pasta with tuna or smoked mackerel; seafood pasta; stir-fried vegetables and rice noodles; Udon noodle soup.	Pasta with creamy sauce, such as carbonara; beef lasagne; pasta with cheese sauce; noodles with sweet and sour sauce.
 Vegetable dishes	Vegetable-stuffed peppers; stir-fried vegetables; tofu; vegetable soup; steamed vegetables with rice; ratatouille; vegetable kebabs; boiled potatoes.	Vegetable pizza; spring rolls; vegetable samosas; vegetable pasty; roast, sautéed, or mashed potatoes cooked with oil or butter; chips; fried rice.
 Desserts	Fresh fruit salad; fruit sorbet; small portion of dessert, or one portion shared with a friend.	Tiramisu; cheesecake; chocolate mousse; kulfi; ice cream; sauces based on cream or alcohol.

Weight and diabetes

Maintaining a healthy weight is one of the most important steps you can take to manage your diabetes. Being overweight can raise your blood glucose level and cause high blood pressure, increasing your risk of heart and circulatory problems. Where on your body you carry any excess weight is also important.

Why weight matters

Your weight can influence how easy it is to manage your diabetes and can make a difference to the type and dose of any medication you take. Being overweight makes managing your blood glucose level, blood pressure, and cholesterol more difficult and increases the risk of heart disease. Keeping your weight within the ideal range for your height or, if you need to, losing some weight, has many health benefits. To assess whether you are overweight you need to measure your body mass index (BMI), which is a ratio of your weight to your height. To work out your BMI, you can either use a chart (see opposite) or calculate it by dividing your weight in kilograms by the square of your height in metres. For example, if you weigh 65 kg and are 1.7 m tall, your BMI is $65 \div (1.7 \times 1.7)$, which equals 22.5, a figure that puts you in the healthy weight category (BMI 18.5–24.9).

Weight and type 2 diabetes

You are more likely to develop type 2 diabetes if you are overweight because this can make your cells resistant to insulin. Four out of five people with type 2 are overweight. If you are overweight, even losing a small amount will make it easier to manage your blood glucose level, lower your blood pressure and

cholesterol, and prevent or delay the onset of future complications, such as heart disease (see pp.192–195). You are also likely to need a lower dose of tablets or less insulin. Losing more weight may help you reverse your type 2 diabetes (see pp.22–23).

CAUSES OF WEIGHT GAIN AND WEIGHT LOSS

Weight loss

Weight gain

Weight loss	Weight gain
Common in people with type 1 diabetes when first diagnosed. Starting treatment with insulin will help you to regain lost weight.	Can be a side effect of some tablets for type 2 diabetes (see pp.58–59). Discuss possible alternatives with your health professional.
May occur gradually with type 2 diabetes if blood glucose levels are consistently high: this means your body is not using glucose properly for energy and instead is using fat from stores in your muscles and beneath your skin.	Having extra snacks for fear of hypos when you use insulin or insulin-stimulating medication.

Taking more insulin than you need; this can cause you to eat more, leading to more storage of fat. |
| May be an effect of other conditions, possibly related to your diabetes, that produce weight loss. One such example is an overactive thyroid. | Eating too many calories, for a variety of reasons, including as an effect of comfort eating. If this applies to you, your health professional can help with practical and emotional support. |
| Not taking enough insulin in order to prevent weight gain, developing an eating disorder, or emotional distress. | Becoming less active because you are physically unable to take any exercise or find it difficult to fit physical activity into your day. |

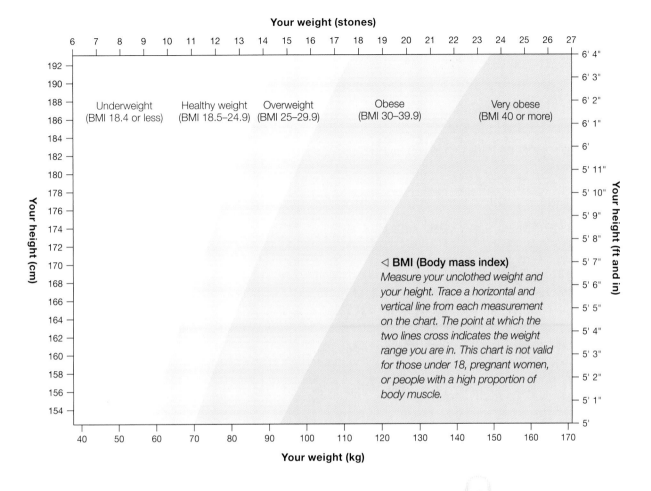

Your weight (stones)

Underweight (BMI 18.4 or less)
Healthy weight (BMI 18.5–24.9)
Overweight (BMI 25–29.9)
Obese (BMI 30–39.9)
Very obese (BMI 40 or more)

Your height (cm)

Your height (ft and in)

◁ **BMI (Body mass index)**
Measure your unclothed weight and your height. Trace a horizontal and vertical line from each measurement on the chart. The point at which the two lines cross indicates the weight range you are in. This chart is not valid for those under 18, pregnant women, or people with a high proportion of body muscle.

Your weight (kg)

Why body shape matters

Body shape is more important than weight itself in terms of your risk of heart disease. If you carry extra fat around your middle rather than around your hips, you have an increased risk of problems.

• Waist circumference: If your waist is more than 102 cm (for a man) or 88 cm (for a woman), you are higher risk of heart and circulation problems.

• Waist-to-hip ratio: Divide your waist measurement by your hip measurement. If the result is more than 0.9 (for a man) or more than 0.85 (for a woman) your risk of developing heart disease is higher.

▷ **Measuring your body**
By taking accurate measurements of your waist and hips you can check your risk of heart and circulation problems. Even if your BMI is in the healthy range, too much fat around your waist indicates that you are at increased risk.

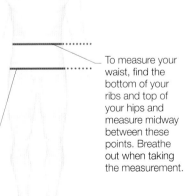

Measure your hips at the widest point

To measure your waist, find the bottom of your ribs and top of your hips and measure midway between these points. Breathe out when taking the measurement.

How to lose weight

The best approach to losing weight – and the way to keep the weight off – is to eat fewer calories and/or be more active. There are several ways of doing this, including calorie counting, intermittent fasting, and low-carbohydrate eating. For any method, planning ahead and finding support will help to keep you motivated.

First steps

If you are overweight, bringing your weight down into the recommended range for your height (see pp.92–93) will be beneficial: your blood glucose level and blood pressure will come down, your blood cholesterol level will improve, and you may well look and feel better. Once you have lost weight, maintaining it within recommended range will help you to keep healthy.

You are more likely to succeed in losing weight if you set yourself practical targets. For example, aim to lose about 0.5–1 kg per week. You may find you lose more weight one week than you do the next. This is normal as your body adjusts to new eating habits. It is important to lose weight gradually: most "quick-fix" diets that produce rapid weight loss are unhealthy, especially if followed long-term, and you are less likely to keep the weight off.

Using a food diary

The first step towards successful weight loss is to look at your eating habits so that you can plan what to do differently. Recording what and when you eat and drink and how you feel can show where you might be taking in excess calories, whether your meals are spread evenly through the day, and whether you are snacking unnecessarily between meals.

When reviewing your food diary, ask yourself the following questions:
- Do I eat high-fat or high-sugar foods at particular times of the day?
- Do I tend to eat in response to my feelings or when I'm bored?
- Do I use ordinary mixers with alcoholic drinks instead of low-calorie versions?
- Do I eat out often and so have less control over what I eat?
- Do I eat very large meals?

If you answered "yes" to any of these questions, you could make changes straight away to help you lose weight.

Making an action plan

When you have decided to lose weight, it is useful to come up with an action plan that is realistic and will work for you. In devising a plan, you may find it helpful to consider the following:
- How much weight would I like to lose?

 KEEPING YOURSELF MOTIVATED

- Empty your fridge and cupboards of tempting high-calorie foods and replace them with lower-calorie alternatives.

- Keep a record of your successes. Don't focus only on your weight – also include extra activity and how often you have resisted temptation.

- Put encouraging notes or inspirational pictures on your fridge and cupboard doors to remind you what you are aiming for.

- Ask for the support of a friend or family member who will give you encouragement when you need it.

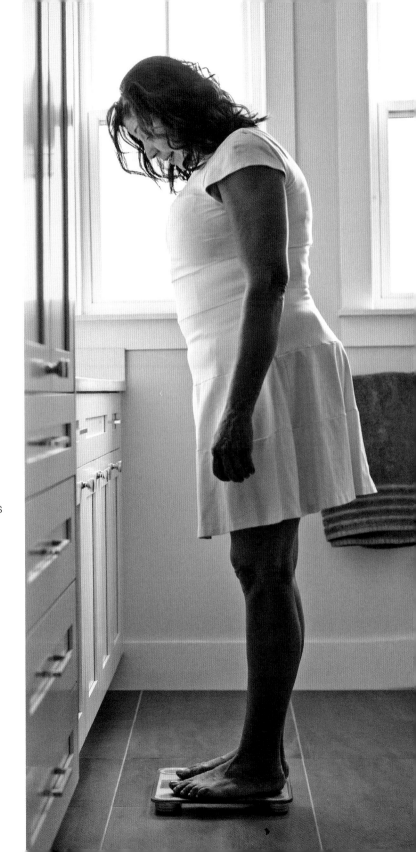

▷ **Checking progress**
*When trying to lose weight, weighing
yourself regularly will enable you to
assess your progress. For accurate
results, weigh yourself with the same
scales at the same time each day, and
wear the same or no clothes every time.*

• What specific changes am I going
to make to what or when I eat?

• What changes am I going to make
to increase my physical activity?

• How will I change my normal routine
to fit in these changes?

• How will I find out how much weight
I have lost each week?

• How will I motivate myself to achieve
my weekly targets?

• Who will I ask to help me stay
motivated?

• What will I do on the occasions when
I can't do what I have decided?

• When will I start my weight-loss plan?

Work out ways to bring about changes
and deal with challenges, and write them
down. For example, you could write
reminders to yourself to eat a healthy
snack before going out for a meal, to
avoid being too hungry to resist higher-
calorie foods, or to keep fruit or unsalted
nuts in your bag or car; or you could
make a list of enjoyable activities that
will distract you from thoughts of food
when you are tempted to snack.

Once you feel confident that your
weight-loss plan is achievable, you might
find it helpful to take time to list strategies
for overcoming temptation when your
resistance is low. Keep the list to hand
so that you can refer to it whenever you
need inspiration.

Setting targets

Being realistic about how much weight you're likely to lose will help you avoid feeling discouraged. Ask yourself whether your target is realistically achievable. If it seems over-optimistic, set yourself smaller targets that you can reach quickly and easily. For example, aiming to lose 1 kg by next week is far easier to work towards than a goal of losing 20 kg by next year. All of those single 1-kg weeks will soon add up. Being successful once in doing what you have planned means you are likely to succeed again.

You may also find it useful to set targets related to food intake rather than weight. For example, if you decide to cut out or cut down on certain foods during the week, you will still feel positive at the end of the week when you have achieved your targets – even if your weight loss is a little slower than you would like.

Calorie counting

The number of kilocalories (usually shortened to calories) or kilojoules listed for foods and drinks tells you their energy content. To maintain a healthy weight, you need to eat around 2,000 calories per day if you are a woman, and 2,500 calories per day if you are a man.

To lose around 0.5 kg per week simply by eating less, you need to reduce the number of calories you consume by 500 a day so that you lose weight by using stored fat for energy instead of calories from food. Fat contains double

---

UNDERSTANDING A FOOD LABEL

Labels on packets and tins of food have useful information on the energy value (calorie content) of foods, as well as the individual components. Food labels typically show the amount of fat (saturated and unsaturated), carbohydrate, protein, fibre, and salt (written as sodium) per 100 g as well as per portion. Knowing how each item listed on a label affects your health will help you choose foods that can help you lose weight and also help you to manage your blood glucose levels.

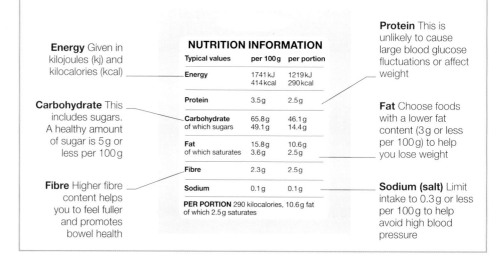

Energy Given in kilojoules (kj) and kilocalories (kcal)

Carbohydrate This includes sugars. A healthy amount of sugar is 5 g or less per 100 g

Fibre Higher fibre content helps you to feel fuller and promotes bowel health

Protein This is unlikely to cause large blood glucose fluctuations or affect weight

Fat Choose foods with a lower fat content (3 g or less per 100 g) to help you lose weight

Sodium (salt) Limit intake to 0.3 g or less per 100 g to help avoid high blood pressure

NUTRITION INFORMATION

Typical values	per 100 g	per portion
Energy	1741 kJ 414 kcal	1219 kJ 290 kcal
Protein	3.5 g	2.5 g
Carbohydrate of which sugars	65.8 g 49.1 g	46.1 g 14.4 g
Fat of which saturates	15.8 g 3.6 g	10.6 g 2.5 g
Fibre	2.3 g	2.5 g
Sodium	0.1 g	0.1 g

PER PORTION 290 kilocalories, 10.6 g fat of which 2.5 g saturates

the calories of the same weight of carbohydrate, so cutting back on fats in your diet is a good start. However, you still need a variety of food types to supply all the nutrients you need, so excluding an entire type of food, such as carbohydrate or protein, is not a healthy approach. Cutting out carbohydrate is particularly unwise as it is your main source of energy. It is best to eat smaller portions of different types of foods, making sure that you include all the food groups across the day.

YOUR MINDSET

Losing weight is as much a mental as a physical challenge. You are more likely to succeed if you plan how to manage when it's hard to resist temptation, you're not in control of what to eat, or you're feeling unhappy about your progress. Build up a non-judgemental support network of family and friends, others trying to lose weight, health professionals or coaches, and diabetes-related or general weight-loss groups and organizations.

You are much more **likely to succeed** in losing weight if you set yourself **practical, realistic targets**

HIGHER-CALORIE FOOD	LOWER-CALORIE FOOD

 Two slices of deep-dish cheese pizza (170 g) 575 calories ····> Two slices of thin-crust pizza (125 g) 380 calories

 Beef hamburger (90 g) 266 calories ····> Salmon burger (90 g) 185 calories

 Chicken breast with skin (200 g) 330 calories ····> Chicken breast without skin (200 g) 185 calories

 Cheddar cheese (50 g) 215 calories ····> Cottage cheese (50 g) 50 calories

◁ **Food swaps to reduce calories**
You can make simple food swaps on an everyday basis that will reduce your calorie intake and help you lose weight without denying yourself foods you like. Examples of calorie-reducing food swaps are shown here, but you can make your own list by using nutritional data from online or other resources.

PROS AND CONS OF INTERMITTENT FASTING

PROS	CONS
Helps you to feel less restricted than a plan you follow every day, which can feel easier and be motivating.	Feeling hungry can be uncomfortable, especially at the start.
It is effective for fairly rapid weight loss so you see results quickly.	You need to drink more fluids to compensate for the fluids you would otherwise have got from food.
You can be flexible with fasting days and timings.	Your fasting or time-limited days may be inconvenient for work or social reasons.
It can benefit other important aspects of your health, for example lowering blood pressure and cholesterol levels.	Lower-calorie or time-limited eating may not fit well with your diabetes regimen, for example, causing more hypos if you use insulin or insulin-stimulating medication.

How to reduce calorie intake

At first, you may need to refer to a book or website listing the calorie contents of foods and weigh some foods, to work out exactly how many calories you are taking in. You can then use your food diary to identify where extra calories are coming from and decide how to reduce your calorie intake. Knowing how to read the nutritional information on food labels (see p.96) will help you make healthier choices when you are shopping.

Some types of food and drink are deceptive, so you may be consuming them without realizing how many hidden calories they contain. For example, fruit juice is high in sugar; alcohol contains a lot of calories; and some sauces that accompany meals are high in fat.

If you are physically active, you can allow yourself a few more calories and still lose weight: physical activity burns calories while you are doing it as well as raising your metabolic rate (the rate at which your body uses up energy) for a period afterwards.

Intermittent fasting

In this regimen, you reduce your daily calorie total on certain days of the week (for example, from 2,000 calories a day to 1,000 on Mondays and Thursdays or on alternate days), or by creating a daily eating time window (for example, only eating between 10 a.m. and 6 p.m. every day or on certain days). By eating fewer calories at these times, and continuing to follow healthy eating principles (see pp.74–75) at other times, you reduce your overall calorie intake. Fasting can also help you to more easily identify times when you feel hungry or full but needs careful planning when you have diabetes (see panel, opposite).

Low-carbohydrate eating

Reducing carbohydrates can reduce both calories and blood glucose levels. To follow a lower-carbohydrate eating plan, you reduce your portion size of carbohydrates or replace higher-carb foods with lower-carb ones and also eat healthy foods from other groups, such as fat and protein, so that you feel full but avoid being too hungry.

Cutting out carbs completely is not the purpose of low-carbohydrate eating, as you still need other nutrients that carbohydrate foods provide, such as vitamins, iron, and fibre. Like intermittent fasting, lower-carb eating helps you to lose weight by reducing your overall calories so that you use up energy stored as fat. By still eating some carbs each day or meal, you feel less deprived, which in turn makes losing weight feel easier. Low- or lower-carb eating may also help you if you are trying to avoid or reverse type 2 diabetes (see pp.22–23). Whether you have type 1 or type 2 diabetes, you will need to monitor your blood glucose and adjust your diabetes medication or regimen according to your blood glucose level while reducing your carbohydrate foods.

Dieting and ketones

When you restrict your calorie intake, you force your body to burn its fat stores for energy. As part of this process, your body may produce by-products known as ketones, which are excreted from your body in urine.

Producing ketones can be normal if you are losing weight. However, for people with type 1 diabetes, producing ketones when you have a high blood glucose level can be toxic and indicate a dangerous lack of insulin (see p.71).

MANAGING YOUR DIABETES WHEN ON A NEW EATING PLAN

Before you start any new eating plan, you need to think about how to coordinate it with your diabetes management.

- Plan in advance how to manage your blood glucose levels and your use of insulin or other medication.

- If you are not sure how to make changes yourself, work out a plan with a health professional – ideally a registered dietitian.

- Have a short initial trial period of your new eating plan, such as 1–2 weeks, to assess your progress.

- Hypos are a particular risk if you use insulin or insulin-stimulating medication, so monitor your blood glucose carefully several times a day, especially when first reducing your food.

- Drink extra water or low-calorie fluids to keep hydrated.

HIGHER-CARBOHYDRATE FOOD   **LOWER-CARBOHYDRATE SWAP**

Quiche Lorraine (100g)
20g carbohydrate
270 calories

Greek salad (140g)
3g carbohydrate
85 calories

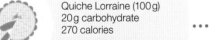
Spaghetti carbonara (260g)
40g carbohydrate
445 calories

Cashew and vegetable stir fry (300g)
11g carbohydrate
310 calories

Sweetcorn (80g)
11g carbohydrate
60 calories

Sugar snap peas (80g)
4g carbohydrate
25 calories

Glazed ring doughnut (100g)
39g carbohydrate
250 calories

Pancake (43g) with maple syrup (8g)
17g carbohydrate
110 calories

◁ **Food swaps to reduce carbohydrates**
You can eat less carbohydrate and fewer calories by reducing the portion size of your meal or by swapping higher-carbohydrate foods for lower-carbohydrate ones that are lower in calories but still give you a range of nutrients.

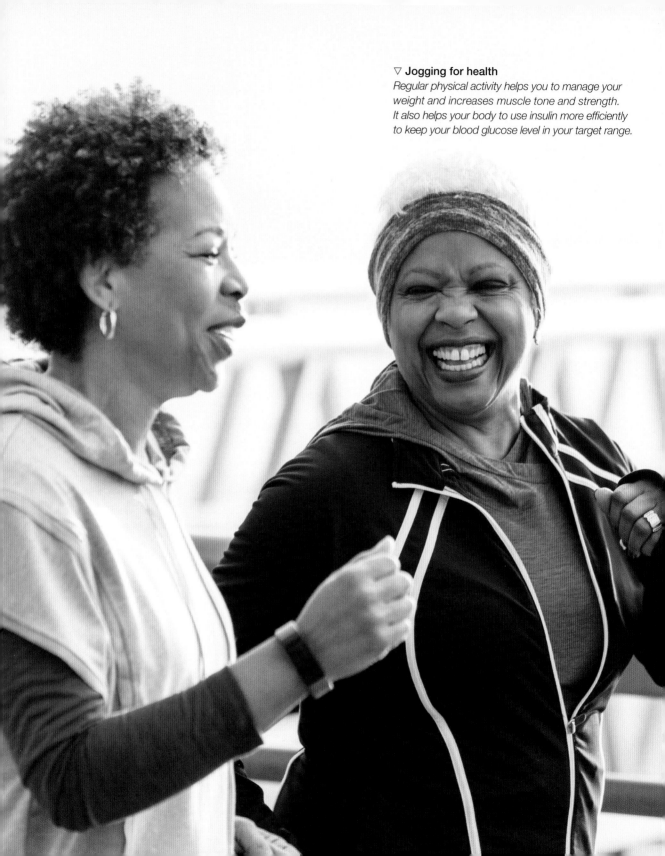

▽ **Jogging for health**
Regular physical activity helps you to manage your weight and increases muscle tone and strength. It also helps your body to use insulin more efficiently to keep your blood glucose level in your target range.

Physical activity

Having a reasonably active lifestyle makes a huge difference to your general health and wellbeing as well as to your diabetes. Whether you want to walk, dance, or run a marathon is up to you: if you are moderately active on a regular and long-term basis you will feel the benefits.

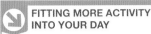

FITTING MORE ACTIVITY INTO YOUR DAY

- Walk or cycle short distances instead of driving.
- Get off the bus one stop earlier and walk the rest of the way.
- Use the stairs instead of the lift if you are only going up one or two floors.
- Park your car a little further from your destination.
- Incorporate a short walk into your daily routine, perhaps after lunch or in the evening.
- Do some extra gardening or housework.

Benefits of activity

Being physically active is good for everyone but is especially important when you have diabetes. It strengthens your heart, muscles, and bones, improves circulation, and helps you to manage your weight. Being active also makes you feel fitter, healthier, and happier, partly because your body is working more efficiently and partly because activity raises levels of brain chemicals that influence your mood. If you are prone to anxiety or depression, physical activity can help prevent or reduce this.

When you have diabetes, as little as 150 minutes of moderate activity a week can help to regulate your blood glucose level and reduce the risk of developing long-term complications. If you have type 2 diabetes, regular activity helps to reduce insulin resistance, which helps the insulin still produced by your own body to work more efficiently. This may delay the need for increases in the dosage of your tablets or mean that you do not need to start having insulin injections. If you have type 1 diabetes, being more active helps the injected insulin to work more efficiently, as well as having the health benefits described above.

How fit are you?

Before you start regular activity, check your existing fitness and activity levels. Can you climb two flights of stairs without shortness of breath or tiredness in your legs? Do you normally take the stairs rather than the escalator or lift? Would you walk for a 10-minute journey rather than drive? Can you have a conversation during light to moderate activity, such as walking? Do you do 150 minutes of moderate physical activity that makes you sweat and breathe harder every week? If you answered "no" to any of the questions above, you could benefit from being more active (see pp.102–105).

CALORIES USED BY EVERYDAY ACTIVITIES

Day-to-day activities use a surprising number of calories. Doing daily chores as part of your activity programme is a good way of boosting your calorie expenditure.

ACTIVITY	CALORIES PER 30 MINUTES
Climbing stairs	330
Gardening, digging	240
House cleaning	120
Gardening, weeding	105
Ironing	60

Being more active

With planning and encouragement, you can find ways to enjoy a more active life and become fitter and healthier. Find activities that you like doing and get started by building up slowly and developing a routine. Whichever type of diabetes you have, being more active will improve your general health as well as your blood glucose levels.

Getting started

Having diabetes places no restrictions on the type of physical activity you can do. However, if you haven't been active for some time, your best route is to start with any form of gentle activity, assess its effect on your blood glucose level, and adjust your diabetes care accordingly. You can then build up your fitness programme gradually.

Once your body is used to regular activity you should aim to be active enough to feel warm and slightly out of breath. If you can sing while you are active, you could probably work harder; if you feel you are gasping for breath, slow down and get your breath back. Your activity is too hard if you experience any pain.

Physical activity doesn't necessarily mean competitive sports or weight training. It also includes less vigorous pursuits, such as walking, gardening, or housework. Doing something moderately energetic (for example, brisk walking, water aerobics, or riding a bike) for 30 minutes a day, five times a week (or at least 150 minutes a week), will improve your fitness and help you to manage your blood glucose more easily.

Building up your fitness

Fitness is a combination of stamina, flexibility, and strength. If your aim is to improve your fitness, you need to do regular activity that makes your heart and lungs work harder (to build stamina), improves mobility in your joints (to increase flexibility), and develops your muscle strength.

If you want to lose weight, you may find that gentle activity, combined with changes in your food intake, is enough to achieve this. If this doesn't work, you will need to burn more calories to lose weight. You could do this by increasing the intensity of the activity, by doing it more often or for longer, or by choosing

---

↘ GETTING AND STAYING MOTIVATED

- Set realistic goals and gradually make them more challenging.

- Keep a record of your activity plan and your exercise programme. It can help you to see what you have achieved. It can also help you identify where your plan worked and where it might need to be changed.

- If a situation occurs to prevent you from being active, such as illness or a change in your working hours, don't feel that a lapse means you have failed – revise your plan and get back to your activity as soon as you can.

- Devise a reward system for yourself to celebrate your success at regular intervals.

- Consider whether a fitness tracker or app could help. These can be set to your personal goals and prompt you to be active regularly.

- Keep your activity kit readily available, so that you can take advantage of unexpected opportunities to be active.

FITNESS BENEFITS OF DIFFERENT ACTIVITIES

When selecting a new activity, you can choose which aspect of your health and fitness to work on: weight loss, stamina, flexibility, or strength. The fitness benefits of selected forms of activity are indicated below on a scale of 1 (small) to 5 (excellent).

ACTIVITY	CALORIES PER 30 MINS	STAMINA	FLEXIBILITY	STRENGTH
Aerobics	215	●●●	●●●	●●
Cycling (fast)	280	●●●●	●●●	●●●
Running	245	●●●●	●●	●●
Swimming (fast)	300	●●●●	●●●	●●●●●
Tennis	210	●●●	●●●	●●●
Walking (brisk)	180	●●	●●	●●

an activity that uses more calories. With any type of activity, remember to warm up before and cool down afterwards. Finish by stretching.

If you aren't able to fit in or get to outside activities, you can still build up your fitness at home, for example, by following exercise programmes online, on television or DVD, or in printed media. If you have mobility difficulties, your health professional will be able to help you find a personalized activity programme.

Planning your activity

You may find it helpful to work out an activity plan. The more detailed your plan, the more likely you are to succeed.

• Decide what you want to achieve – for example, do you want to feel healthier or lose weight? Your goal will help you plan which type of activity and how much of it you need to do.
• Choose an activity that you will find enjoyable – you're more likely to find the time to do it.
• Be realistic about how often you will be able to pursue an activity. Will you be able to fit it into your normal day, or will you need to find extra time to do it?
• Consider teaming up with a friend, partner, or family member. This may make getting fit more enjoyable and also give you the encouragement you need to stay active.

Activity and blood glucose

Any physical activity affects your blood glucose level. The effect depends on how intense the type of exercise is and how long you exercise for. If you take insulin or tablets to manage your diabetes and you exercise intensively or for a long period, monitoring your blood glucose level closely will help you take action to prevent a hypo.

How activity affects blood glucose

When you exercise, you need extra energy. Your body gets the energy it needs by converting the glycogen that is stored in your liver and muscles back to glucose. It also gets energy from the fat stored around your body. Gentle activity for 10–30 minutes is unlikely to have much effect on your blood glucose level. However, if you are more vigorous, your blood glucose level will fall because of the extra glucose your muscles are using. When you stop being physically active, your muscles and, to a lesser extent, your liver replace their glycogen stores by taking glucose from the

bloodstream. The longer or more intense the activity, the more glucose is needed to replenish these stores, so your blood glucose level could be affected for several hours afterwards.

Checking your blood glucose

If you are starting physical activity for the first time, use your blood glucose readings to check the effect that everyday activities, such as shopping and gardening, have on it. That will give baseline information against which you can assess the effect of your new physical activity. If you already do some regular physical activity that is not very

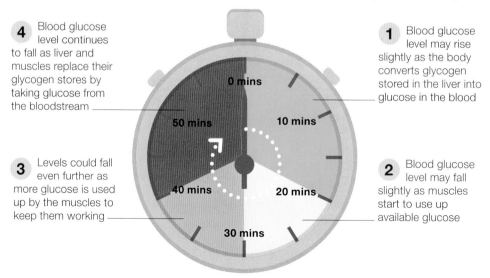

▷ **Impact of activity on blood glucose**
If you are moderately active for 30 minutes or more, your blood glucose level changes throughout the activity. The more intense or long-lasting the activity, the greater the impact on your blood glucose.

4 Blood glucose level continues to fall as liver and muscles replace their glycogen stores by taking glucose from the bloodstream

3 Levels could fall even further as more glucose is used up by the muscles to keep them working

1 Blood glucose level may rise slightly as the body converts glycogen stored in the liver into glucose in the blood

2 Blood glucose level may fall slightly as muscles start to use up available glucose

0 mins
10 mins
20 mins
30 mins
40 mins
50 mins

If you are **active** for more than **an hour**, it is advisable to **check** your **blood glucose** level in the **middle** of your activity

strenuous, note what effect that has on your blood glucose level and then compare it with the effect of more vigorous activity.

If you take insulin-stimulating medication or insulin, check your blood glucose level before and after activity, and again a few hours later. If you are active for more than an hour, check your blood glucose in the middle of the activity as well.

▷ **Keeping track of blood glucose**
You will need to monitor your blood glucose level before and after exercise so that you know the effect of exercise and whether you need a snack to prevent a hypo.

BEING PHYSICALLY ACTIVE SAFELY

Any physical activity, but especially prolonged or strenuous activity, can cause changes in your blood glucose level.

- Keep sugary food or drinks available in case your blood glucose level starts to fall.

- Take your blood glucose monitoring equipment with you if you plan to be active for an hour or more – you may need to do a check.

- Tell someone where you are going and what time you expect to be back if you are going out for a long walk, run, or cycle ride.

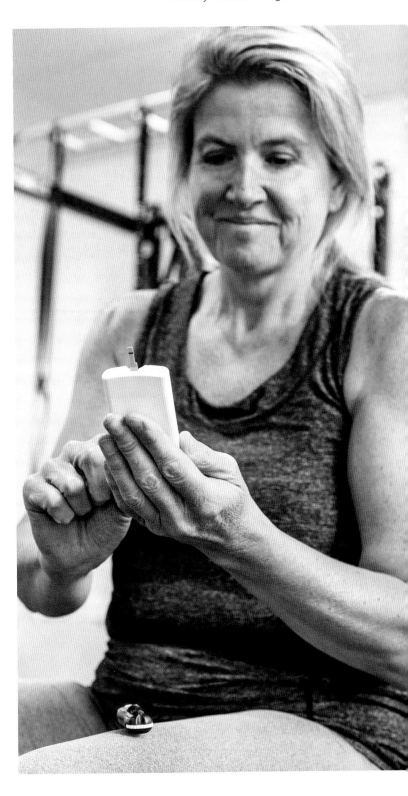

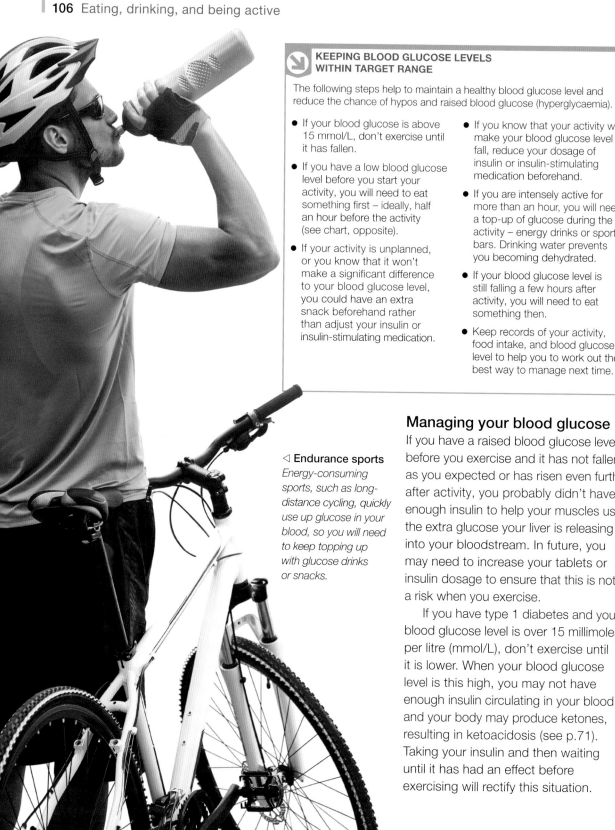

> ### ⬋ KEEPING BLOOD GLUCOSE LEVELS WITHIN TARGET RANGE
>
> The following steps help to maintain a healthy blood glucose level and reduce the chance of hypos and raised blood glucose (hyperglycaemia).
>
> - If your blood glucose is above 15 mmol/L, don't exercise until it has fallen.
> - If you have a low blood glucose level before you start your activity, you will need to eat something first – ideally, half an hour before the activity (see chart, opposite).
> - If your activity is unplanned, or you know that it won't make a significant difference to your blood glucose level, you could have an extra snack beforehand rather than adjust your insulin or insulin-stimulating medication.
>
> - If you know that your activity will make your blood glucose level fall, reduce your dosage of insulin or insulin-stimulating medication beforehand.
> - If you are intensely active for more than an hour, you will need a top-up of glucose during the activity – energy drinks or sports bars. Drinking water prevents you becoming dehydrated.
> - If your blood glucose level is still falling a few hours after activity, you will need to eat something then.
> - Keep records of your activity, food intake, and blood glucose level to help you to work out the best way to manage next time.

◁ **Endurance sports**
Energy-consuming sports, such as long-distance cycling, quickly use up glucose in your blood, so you will need to keep topping up with glucose drinks or snacks.

Managing your blood glucose

If you have a raised blood glucose level before you exercise and it has not fallen as you expected or has risen even further after activity, you probably didn't have enough insulin to help your muscles use the extra glucose your liver is releasing into your bloodstream. In future, you may need to increase your tablets or insulin dosage to ensure that this is not a risk when you exercise.

If you have type 1 diabetes and your blood glucose level is over 15 millimoles per litre (mmol/L), don't exercise until it is lower. When your blood glucose level is this high, you may not have enough insulin circulating in your blood and your body may produce ketones, resulting in ketoacidosis (see p.71). Taking your insulin and then waiting until it has had an effect before exercising will rectify this situation.

EATING TO MANAGE BLOOD GLUCOSE BEFORE ACTIVITY

Depending on your blood glucose level, you may need to eat a snack before starting activity or, if your blood glucose is very high, wait until it is lower. The examples here are based on the intensity and duration of your intended activity, together with your pre-activity blood glucose level. Ask your health professional for personalized advice.

TYPE AND DURATION OF ACTIVITY	BLOOD GLUCOSE BEFORE ACTIVITY (MMOL/L)	EXAMPLES OF WHAT TO EAT 30 MINUTES BEFORE ACTIVITY
GENTLE: Walking or cycling for less than 30 minutes	5 or less	1 slice of bread or 1 piece of fruit, such as an apple
	Any level above 5	Nothing
MODERATE: Playing golf, leisurely cycling, playing tennis, or swimming for 1 hour	5 or less	1 slice of bread plus 1 piece of fruit, such as an apple
	5–9	1 slice of bread plus 1 piece of fruit, such as an apple
	9–15	Nothing
	Above 15	Activity not advised until blood glucose level is lower. Risk of ketones in type 1 diabetes.
INTENSE: Playing football or tennis for 2 hours. Vigorously cycling or swimming for more than 1 hour	5 or less	2 slices of bread plus 1 piece of fruit, such as an apple
	5–9	1 slice of bread plus 1 piece of fruit, such as an apple
	9–15	1 slice of bread or 1 piece of fruit, such as an apple
	Above 15	Activity not advised until blood glucose level is lower. Risk of ketones in type 1 diabetes.

Prolonged or strenuous activity

If you take insulin or insulin-stimulating medication and are active for 2 hours or more, you will need to pay even closer attention to your blood glucose level, including for up to about 24 hours after you have finished. This is because your blood glucose level might take this long to return to normal as your body gradually replaces the glucose stores in your muscles. Regular blood glucose checks are essential during this period and, if necessary, you may also need to take action to reduce the chance of having a hypo.

If you want to increase your muscle bulk or are training for a specific event, your exercise programme needs to be tailored to your needs. Dealing with endurance sports and diabetes is a specialized area and you may need advice from your health professional.

If your **blood glucose level is** over 15 mmol/L, wait until it is lower **before you exercise**

FOOT CARE

Many types of physical activity involve putting extra pressure on your feet. Wear comfortable, well-fitting shoes that do not rub and make sure that they are appropriate for the type of activity you do. Always check your feet carefully for blisters and any other damage both before and after activity (see pp.122–123). If you do develop blisters or damage the skin of your feet, you will need to ensure they are treated immediately. You may need to avoid activity that may potentially cause further damage until the blisters or skin have completely healed.

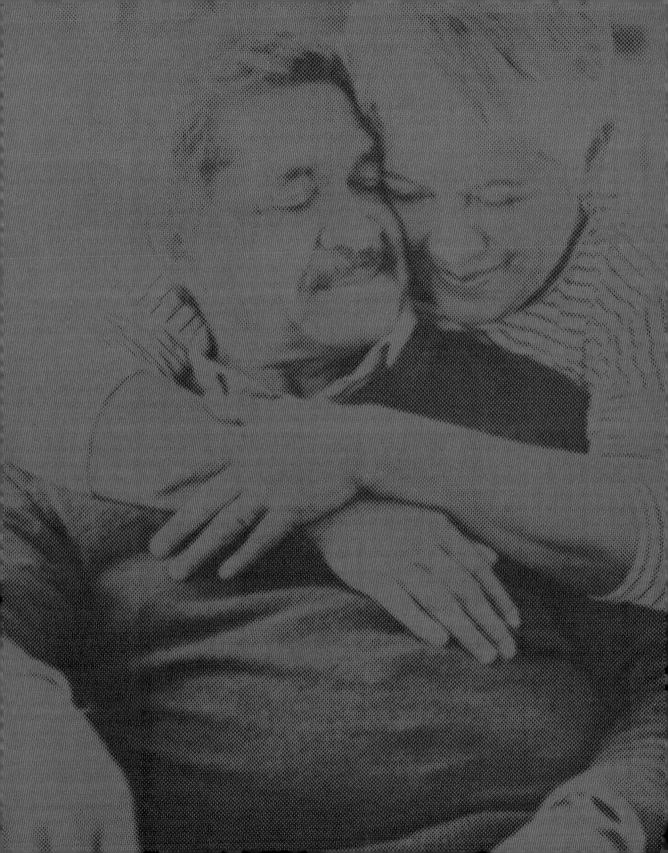

Living with diabetes

Managing your emotions

When you have any type of diabetes, it is normal for it to affect you emotionally as well as physically. Being aware of your feelings, learning to cope with them, and finding support are all just as important in managing your diabetes as the medical aspects.

Recognizing the emotional effects of diabetes

When you are first diagnosed with diabetes, you may experience shock, surprise, anger, fear, or even relief at knowing the cause of health problems you may have been experiencing. Individual reactions can vary greatly – the important thing to know is that it's normal to have an emotional response.

As you become accustomed to knowing you have diabetes and more familiar with managing it, your feelings are likely to change. Discussing your emotional responses, as well as your medical treatment, with your healthcare professionals will help you to become more confident in managing your diabetes. Your feelings may also have a direct physical effect. For example, stress, excitement, or anxiety may affect your blood glucose due to hormones such as adrenaline and cortisol that are released at such times. Learning how to recognize and deal with these effects is also part of managing your diabetes, which is why it's important to discuss your emotions in your regular health reviews with healthcare professionals.

Dealing with the emotional effects of diabetes

Identifying how you feel and whether these feelings are affecting the way you look after your diabetes is a useful first step in dealing with your emotional responses. You could do this in various ways, for example, by talking about them with your family or friends or simply writing them down.

Recognizing that it is understandable to have negative feelings about diabetes can help you to realize that you don't need to feel guilty about these feelings or think that you are failing. Being aware of your feelings also means you will notice if you are losing interest in managing your diabetes. If this persists, ask your health professional for ideas to help.

Getting support

Feeling as though you are not alone with your diabetes can help you to cope with the emotions it brings. In particular, peer

▽ **Professional support**
Your healthcare professional can give you advice and support about emotional issues as well as the more medical aspects of managing your diabetes.

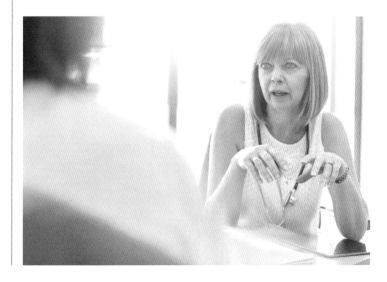

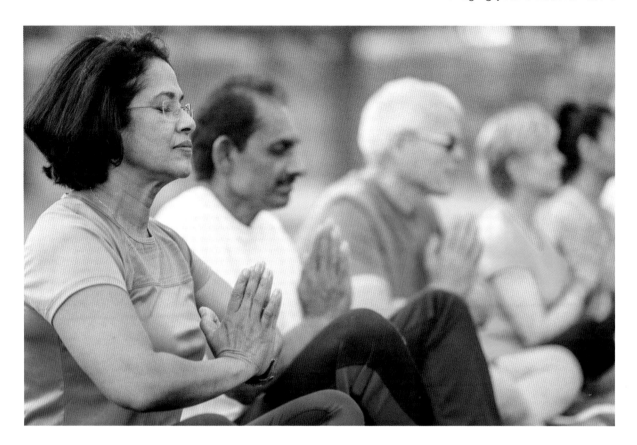

support from other people living with diabetes can be very helpful. You can connect with them in person, through local peer support groups, national diabetes organization meetings and conferences, or online and social media. Your diabetes health professionals can also help you find sources of support, and, if necessary, arrange for additional professional help if you are experiencing more serious psychological problems (see pp.176–179).

Diabetes-related distress and burnout

Sometimes, the relentless day-to-day management of your diabetes can become a burden and you may feel overwhelmed by the demands of living with a condition that never goes away. You may start to take less care of yourself, for example, by paying less attention to your diabetes. Commonly known as diabetes burnout, there are things you can do to deal with it:

● Try to identify any specific concerns you have and then find out if these are justified, for example, your personal risk of long-term complications.

● Consider ways to reduce the physical demands of managing your diabetes. For example, if you use the fingerprick method to check your blood glucose, you could try a flash monitor (see p.35 and p.37).

● Practising progressive relaxation, deep breathing exercises, or mindfulness regularly every day can help you to feel less stressed and more in control.

△ **Reducing stress**
Regular relaxation exercises can help to reduce stress. This, in turn, may help you to feel more in control and may also reduce stress hormones, such as adrenaline, which can impact your blood glucose.

Work*

With diabetes, you can do almost any type of work, even being a prime minister or an Olympic athlete. With rare exceptions, having diabetes will not prevent you from getting a job or keeping your existing one, and there are many ways you can adapt your regimen to minimize any problems. If you do experience difficulties, information, help, and support are available from various sources.

Applying for jobs

You do not need to tell a prospective employer about your diabetes, nor are they legally allowed to ask you about your health. However, you could decide to be open about your diabetes and how you manage it, as a way of showing you look after your health. If you do apply for a job that has restrictions for safety reasons – for example, in the emergency services – you may have to declare your diabetes. In the UK, the armed forces are by law not open to people with diabetes, but there are very few other blanket bans like this in place.

Managing your diabetes at work

Your decision to tell or not tell your employer about your diabetes may depend on what type of diabetes you have and what effect it will have on your job. For example, if you need to take insulin or insulin-stimulating medication and you work shifts involving driving or using machinery, this will have more implications for your medication

timings and safety if you experience a hypo (see pp.62–67) than if you work more regular hours in an office. Your employment contract and your employer's health and safety policy will specify what information you need to give and to whom. If you are at risk of a hypo, telling your manager and/or a first aider about your diabetes and its treatment is advisable so that someone can help if you do have a hypo.

Under UK law, diabetes can be considered to be a disability. This means that employers need to make reasonable adjustments to accommodate what you need to do to look after your diabetes. For example, you may need to work in a different area, have breaks at specific times, or time off for diabetes health appointments or education.

In general, looking after your diabetes will contribute to your health, which will help you do your job as well as possible. You can manage your diabetes as discreetly or openly as you wish. It is sensible to devise a plan for your medication, eating, and blood glucose monitoring to fit in with your routine, and your health professional can help you with this. They can also help you adapt your regimen, if necessary, to make life at work easier. For example, you might

However busy your job, it is important to care for your diabetes in order to feel well

consider using a flash monitor (see pp.35 and 37) to make blood glucose checking quicker, or a longer-acting type of medication (see pp.44–45 and 58–59) so that you don't have to take doses at work. Thinking about how to avoid and treat hypos and what equipment to store at work is also helpful.

Dealing with problems

If your diabetes does start to cause problems at work – for example, if you develop a complication that makes you less able to do your job – you need to inform your employer so that you can discuss possibilities for the future. If you feel you need support in this situation, your health professional will help.

Many employers are understanding and flexible in relation to diabetes-related needs, but in some situations you may feel you are experiencing discrimination because of your diabetes. If you suspect this is the case:

• Obtain evidence of the issue, in writing if possible.
• Consult the health and equality policies of the company you work for.
• Ask your health professional for advice and support.
• Seek help from national diabetes organizations.
• If necessary, obtain expert legal advice, for example, from an advice centre or employment lawyer.

▽ **Managing work and diabetes**
Caring for your diabetes will help you perform well at work. Whether you tell your colleagues about your condition is your choice, but if you are at risk of hypos, it can be helpful if they know what to do.

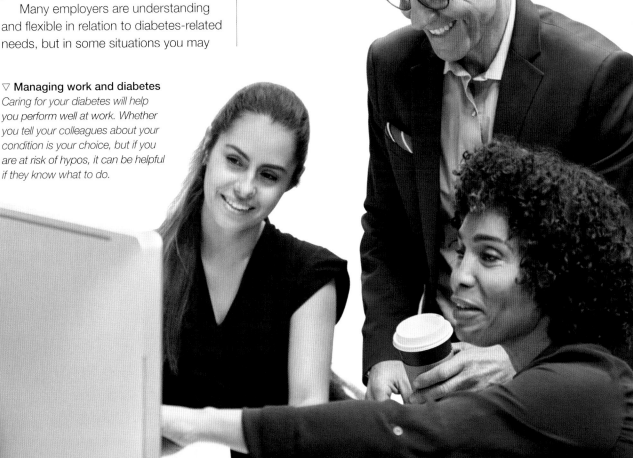

Driving

Most people with diabetes can obtain a licence for most types of vehicle and can carry on driving. However, there are special precautions you should take when you have diabetes and drive, and there are also particular regulations concerning driving and diabetes that you need to be aware of.

▽ **Driving and diabetes**

Taking a little extra time and care with your diabetes when driving will make your journeys safer (see opposite).

How diabetes may affect driving

An episode of hypoglycaemia (see pp.62–67) can seriously impair your ability to drive safely so it is vital to take precautions to avoid one. You should also ensure that your vision is good enough to drive safely (see pp.182–183). If you have nerve damage (neuropathy, see pp.188–189), it is important that this does not compromise safe driving.

Rules and regulations

If you have any type of diabetes, you need to inform your insurance company. However, an insurance company cannot refuse you insurance or increase your premium unless it has evidence that you are a higher-risk driver. If you take insulin, you need to inform the relevant authorities* as soon as possible after starting treatment. If you take other

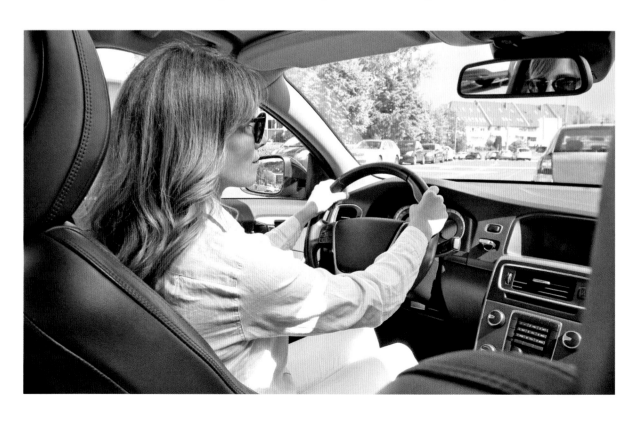

medication for your diabetes, you do not need to inform the authorities if you have full hypoglycaemia awareness.

If you take insulin, your driving licence will be granted on the basis of your risk of hypoglycaemia or whether you have any long-term complications. You will need to provide the authorities with details of your condition and contact details for your doctor or healthcare professional. For certain categories of vehicles, such as passenger-carrying vehicles or large goods vehicles, you must inform the authorities of any medication you take. They will give you more information about the health checks you need. If you are in any doubt about the rules and regulations and how they may affect you, speak to your healthcare professional and/or contact the relevant authorities.

Safe driving

The most potentially serious risk when driving is having a hypo. Not only are you at risk of having an accident, but you could also lose your licence while your hypo awareness is checked.

You are at risk of having a hypo only if you use insulin or insulin-stimulating medication to manage your diabetes. In either case, you must take special care to ensure you are fit to drive before starting a journey, and that you check your blood glucose level frequently during a trip (see chart, below). If you know that you don't experience warning signs of a hypo or if you have had a severe hypo while awake during the past 12 months, you must not drive; in this situation, you need to inform the authorities, and follow their procedures.

SAFE DRIVING CHECKLIST

 Check your blood glucose level before you drive, however short the trip. Only drive if your blood glucose is in the recommended range and above 5 mmol/L.

 Do not delay meals or snacks, or taking your scheduled medication because you are driving. If necessary, stop and eat or take your medication.

 Do not drive if your blood glucose is below 5 mmol/L – you are at risk of a hypo. Eat something if it is 4–5 mmol/L or treat a hypo if it is below 4 mmol/L, and wait 45 minutes before driving.

 Keep supplies of food and drink to treat a hypo where you can reach them easily in the car (not in the boot).

 Stop at least every 2 hours during a long journey and check your blood glucose.

 Take blood glucose monitoring equipment (meter, lancing device, lancets, and strips) with you, even if you use a continuous or flash monitor.

 If you have a hypo while driving, stop the car, turn off the ignition, move to the passenger seat, and treat the hypo. Wait until 45 minutes after your blood glucose has risen above 4 mmol/L and you are feeling well before driving again.

 Carry diabetes identification, your driving licence, your insurance documents, and a mobile phone.

Holidays and travel

When you are away from home, a different environment or routine is likely to affect your diabetes management. For example, long-distance travel, changes in temperature, and different foods, drinks, or activities can all affect your blood glucose. But by planning ahead, you can help to avoid potential problems.

Before you go

Check that your travel insurance covers diabetes and diabetes-related problems while you are away – including any hospital stay – and for your return journey. You should take more than enough diabetes equipment and medication for your trip, because it may be difficult to find replacements at short notice, even within your own country.

If you will be flying, ask your health professional for a letter stating that you have diabetes, what medication and equipment you will be carrying, and explaining that they must be kept in your hand luggage. When packing, split your diabetes supplies in separate bags in case one gets lost or separated from you. If you use an insulin pump, flash monitor, or continuous glucose monitor, you should not be screened by an X-ray or other security scanner, so before you travel, contact your airline and the airports you will be travelling through about special security arrangements.

Looking after your equipment and medication

All of your equipment and medicines should be stored in a cool, dry place. Unopened insulin bottles, cartridges, or disposable injection devices should be kept in a fridge at a temperature of 2–8°C. If you don't have access to a fridge or are travelling long haul, use a cool bag or flask. If you are flying, keep your insulin in your hand luggage – it can freeze in the hold of a plane. The insulin you are currently using will be safe at a temperature of up to 25°C for up to a month, provided you keep it out of direct sunlight. In higher temperatures, you will need to keep it cool. In cold climates, you need to keep your insulin above 2°C.

Crossing time zones

Travelling across time zones can affect your blood glucose, eating pattern, and the timing of your diabetes medication

THINGS TO PACK

- Insulin or tablets – at least double the supply you need.
- Blood glucose monitoring meter, lancets, and test strips.
- Cool bag or flask if you use insulin.
- Hypo treatments if you need them.
- Back-up insulin pens if you use an insulin pump.
- Identification, including your diabetes ID.
- Information on managing your diabetes when you are unwell.
- Insurance details, and your health professional's contact details.

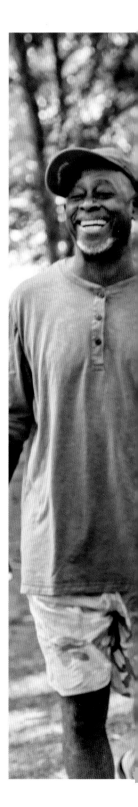

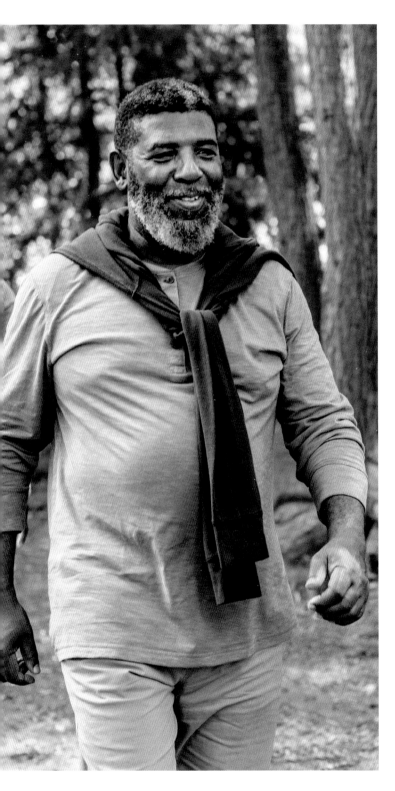

(including insulin). Checking your blood glucose every few hours will enable you to find out whether you need any extra medication or food. It will also alert you to hypos (see pp.62–67) or raised blood glucose (hyperglycaemia, see pp.68–71).

If you are concerned about how crossing times zones may affect your diabetes management, ask your health professional for advice before you travel.

While you are away

In hot conditions, your injected insulin may take effect faster than usual. This may make you prone to hypos, and you might need to reduce your insulin dose or eat extra carbohydrate to compensate. If you become cold, your injected insulin may take longer to work, which may result in hyperglycaemia. Wearing warm clothes and being active can counteract this, so your blood glucose shouldn't rise too high. Trying new foods, drinks, and activities may also affect blood glucose. Checking it frequently will give you the information you need to make the appropriate adjustments to keep your blood glucose in the recommended range. To avoid stomach upsets, which may cause your blood glucose to rise, you should be scrupulous about personal and food hygiene. It is also important to look after your feet. Wear comfortable shoes, never go barefoot, even on the beach, and check your feet frequently.

◁ **New activities**
Having diabetes need not prevent you from enjoying a new activity, such as hiking, on holiday or at any other time. You just have to plan ahead to make sure you can continue to manage your diabetes successfully.

Sex and relationships

Diabetes can affect both you and your partner. It can give rise to conflicting emotions, often due to love, concern, stress, or fear. You may also have practical concerns around contraception, pregnancy, sexual function, and managing your blood glucose levels.

Talking to your partner

You may be wary about discussing your diabetes, especially if you have just been diagnosed or if you have a new partner. However, sharing your feelings, ideally when neither of you is feeling pressured, can help you to understand and support each other. Finding ways of involving your partner if they want to feel included can help. For example, you could invite your partner to your diabetes reviews so that they can get a better understanding of any treatment that you need.

Sex and blood glucose control

Sexual activity can use up a lot of energy, so it should be treated in the same way as other types of physical activity (see pp.104–107). Checking your blood glucose before you have sex and again a few hours later will help you to gauge the effect and decide whether you need to take any measures to prevent a hypo. You may find that you need to either reduce your insulin dose beforehand or eat more to keep your blood glucose in your target range. Bear in mind that your blood glucose level can fall several hours after physical activity.

If you are taking insulin or insulin-stimulating medication, there is a risk that sex could cause hypoglycaemia. Keep some high-glucose snacks or drinks to hand in case you have a hypo, so you can deal with it quickly. Your partner may need to give you a glucagon injection if you become too hypoglycaemic to take action yourself (see pp.66–67).

Sexual function

Problems with sexual performance may have physical or psychological roots. Erectile dysfunction (see p.201) is recognized as a complication of diabetes in men. Sexual function has been less widely researched in women, but it is thought that diabetes can affect a woman's sexual response. Vaginal dryness is a fairly common complaint, while some women might find sex painful, lose interest in sex, or be unable to achieve an orgasm as they used to. If you are experiencing difficulties, you can talk to your health professional about treatment options or counselling.

PREGNANCY AND CONTRACEPTION

It is vital to plan any pregnancy (see pp.132–135) and manage your blood glucose in advance. There is a wide range of contraception methods – for example, condoms and other barrier devices; hormonal methods, such as the contraceptive pill; mechanical methods, such as the IUD; and natural methods that rely on identifying less fertile times in your menstrual cycle. Which method is most suitable for you may depend on your age and on your general and diabetes health. Talk with your health professional about your contraception options.

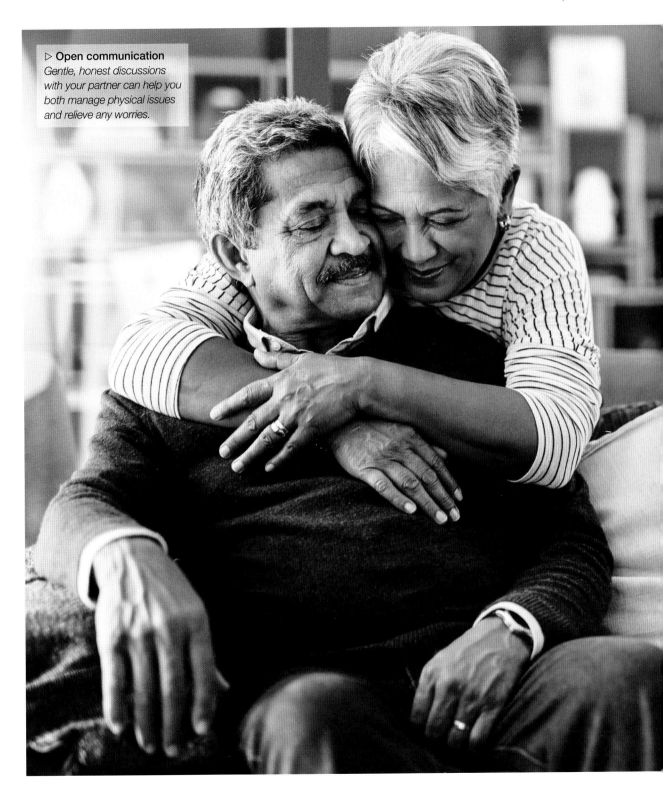

▷ **Open communication**
Gentle, honest discussions with your partner can help you both manage physical issues and relieve any worries.

Keeping healthy*

When you have diabetes, your medical checks and consultations tend to focus on your diabetes, but looking after other aspects of your health is also important. Health screening, regular dental and sight check-ups, keeping your vaccinations up-to-date, staying generally fit, and sleep are all vital to your health with diabetes.

▽ **Dental check-up**
Regular checks of your mouth and teeth by a dentist can help to detect any problems before they become serious, potentially affecting your diabetes management.

Routine health screening

Depending on your age, you will be invited for screening for certain forms of cancer, for example, breast, bowel, and cervical cancer. Attending these is useful, because having diabetes does not mean you are at less risk of these conditions. If your baby or child has diabetes, they will be offered the same developmental checks as for every other child.

Vision and dental check-ups

You will have yearly eye checks for retinopathy (see p.180) because you have diabetes. These do not check your general vision, so regular eye tests are also important – for example, to check for problems such as glaucoma, shortsightednes, and longsightedness and, if necessary, to prescribe glasses or contact lenses to correct your vision.

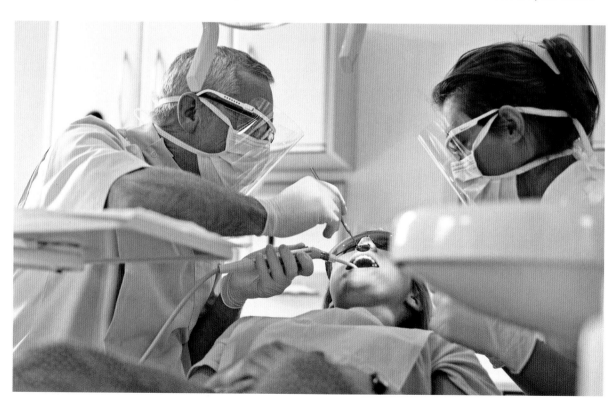

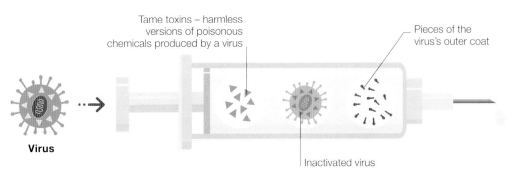

▷ **Vaccines**
Vaccines are made up of an inactivated version of a virus or toxin, or pieces of a virus. They work by priming your immune system, so that it is ready to destroy a real viral infection.

Virus

Tame toxins – harmless versions of poisonous chemicals produced by a virus

Pieces of the virus's outer coat

Inactivated virus

Regular dental check-ups are particularly important if you have diabetes, because the condition increases the risk of problems such as gum disease. Early detection and treatment of such problems can help prevent severe infections and possible loss of teeth. In addition, if you develop a dental problem, it can make diabetes harder to manage. As well as regular dental check-ups, looking after your teeth and gums by regular brushing and flossing, and following any advice from your dentist will help to keep your mouth and teeth healthy.

Vaccinations
Vaccination against a range of diseases is offered routinely as part of the national immunization programme, including to people with diabetes. Most vaccinations are offered during childhood or young adulthood, although some, such as shingles, are routinely offered only to older people or special groups, such as pregnant women. When you have diabetes, you are offered additional vaccinations: children and young adults are offered the childhood flu vaccine, and adults of any age with diabetes are offered the flu and pneumococcal vaccines that are usually reserved for those over 65 years. Being vaccinated is advisable for everybody but is particularly valuable for

people with diabetes, as it can prevent you from developing a condition that could make it more difficult to manage your diabetes. If you are travelling to an area where infectious diseases are a risk, ask your healthcare professional about vaccinations for the places you intend to visit and, if necessary, have the recommended vaccines or boosters.

General fitness and strength
For everyone, keeping fit and strong helps overall health. At specific times of life, from middle age onwards (and for women, especially after the menopause) healthy bones and muscles become particularly important in helping to prevent osteoporosis and falls, with their possible negative effect on your blood glucose and its treatment. Physical activity and weight-bearing exercise will help to keep your bones and muscles strong, as will paying attention to your vitamin D intake.

Sleep
Having 7–9 hours of good-quality sleep is linked with your body cells repairing themselves, regulation of your appetite-controlling hormones, and feeling positive and relaxed. These can all have a beneficial effect on your blood glucose level and how you manage it.

Footcare

Over time, diabetes can impair your blood circulation or damage your nerves. Your feet are especially susceptible to problems resulting from poor circulation or nerve damage (see pp.188–191), but by making sure you pay special attention to good footcare, you can reduce the risk of such problems developing.

Routine footcare

Your feet and circulation will be examined at your annual review (see pp.142–143), but between reviews you can establish the habit of cleaning and checking your feet every day. Cut your toenails when necessary. However, if you have reduced feeling or circulation in your feet, check with your health professional that it is still all right for you to cut your own nails. If you are not able to cut your own toenails or check your feet properly yourself, ask somebody to help you or consult a registered podiatrist. You can help to prevent injuries by never walking barefoot – not even in your own home.

When buying footwear, try to choose well-fitting, supportive shoes that have enough room for your toes and do not rub. In particular, avoid pointed shoes and high heels for everyday wear, and do not wear them at all if you have reduced feeling or poor circulation in your feet. It is also wise to avoid wearing tight socks, tights, or stockings that rub or cramp your toes.

Check your footwear daily to ensure that there are no areas that rub and that there are no sharp objects inside the shoe or sticking through the sole. From time to time, check the soles and uppers of your shoes for uneven wear that may indicate particular pressure areas. Make sure you avoid putting your feet directly against a hot radiator, heater, or hot-water bottle, or near an open fire, as you may accidentally burn your feet if loss of sensation means you can't feel the heat.

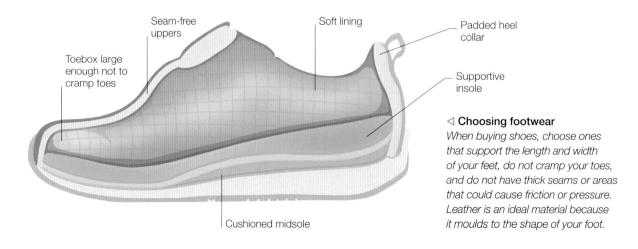

Seam-free uppers

Soft lining

Padded heel collar

Toebox large enough not to cramp toes

Supportive insole

Cushioned midsole

◁ **Choosing footwear**
When buying shoes, choose ones that support the length and width of your feet, do not cramp your toes, and do not have thick seams or areas that could cause friction or pressure. Leather is an ideal material because it moulds to the shape of your foot.

LOOKING AFTER YOUR FEET

A good footcare routine will help you to keep your feet healthy and enable you to notice potential problems early on. Carry out this procedure every day, especially if you have reduced feeling or circulation in your feet. Allow plenty of time so that you can check your feet thoroughly for any injuries or other problems.

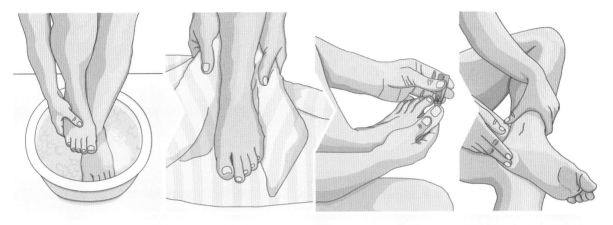

1 Wash or shower your feet daily in warm water, using a mild soap. Avoid soaking your feet for more than 10 minutes, as this can cause wrinkles, which can be damaged easily.

2 Dry your feet carefully, especially between your toes. Then check for any tender areas, bruising, cuts, or hard or cracked skin on the top and on the soles of your feet.

3 Trim your toenails. Cut them to the shape of, and level with, the end of your toe. Don't cut them too short. Don't use sharp instruments on your nails or anywhere else on your feet.

4 Apply an unperfumed moisturizing cream to your feet, paying particular attention to any hard skin on your soles. Avoid using too much between your toes.

Dealing with foot problems

You can treat certain problems yourself, but some common ones, such as corns and calluses, should be dealt with by a health professional. Athlete's foot can be treated at home with an over-the-counter antifungal preparation. Keep the skin clean and dry, especially between your toes. If you have a small blister, do not put pressure on it or pop it. If it does pop, cover it with gauze and check it often to make sure it is healing. Verrucas will eventually clear up without treatment but they may cause pressure points. They should be assessed by a health professional so that you know how to treat them properly.

 GETTING PROFESSIONAL HELP

Many foot problems require professional care, so contact your health professional if you develop any of the conditions below, or if you cannot look after your feet yourself and there is nobody else to help.

- Corns, calluses, or areas of hard or cracked skin.
- Burns or other injuries.
- A sore area that is not healing.
- An ingrowing toenail.
- Bruises or discoloured areas that have no apparent cause.
- Any new loss of feeling in any part of your foot.

Dealing with illness

Diabetes does not make you more prone to common illnesses, but if your blood glucose is consistently high, you may pick up infections more easily or simply feel unwell. Illness can also affect your diabetes, and how well you are able to manage your blood glucose can affect the speed of your recovery.

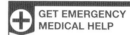

GET EMERGENCY MEDICAL HELP

- If you develop symptoms of diabetic ketoacidosis (DKA): fruity-smelling breath; pain in the abdomen; nausea; vomiting; thirst; frequent passing of urine; deep breathing; high and rising blood glucose level; ketones in blood or urine; confusion.

- If you develop symptoms of hyperosmolar hyperglycaemic state (HHS): nausea; thirst; frequent passing of urine; dry skin; high and rising blood glucose level; confusion.

The effect of illness on your diabetes

Whatever type of diabetes you have, illness is likely to raise your blood glucose, because your body responds to illness by releasing more glucose into the blood and producing stress hormones. These hormones make your natural or injected insulin less efficient, which can cause hyperglycaemia (raised blood glucose) even if you are not eating anything. One of the symptoms of hyperglycaemia is dehydration, which can be worsened by a high body temperature. A sudden, acute illness with vomiting and diarrhoea can cause your diabetes to become unmanageable and can also affect other body processes, which, untreated, may be life-threatening.

Blood glucose levels

You may not be ill often, so you may not remember what effect illness has on your blood glucose. Next time you are unwell, make a note of what you do to manage your blood glucose and keep your notes for reference. When you are ill, continue to take your diabetes medication and check your blood glucose frequently. Keeping your glucose level below 10 millimoles per litre (mmol/L) will

help your recovery. You may need to temporarily increase your dose of medication to achieve this.

Although illness typically causes a rise in blood glucose, occasionally illness can cause it to fall (hypoglycaemia). In this situation, your dose of diabetes medication may need to be reduced, but you need to be careful that this does not make your blood glucose rise too high.

Eating and drinking

Food and drink give your body energy to combat illness and help to limit the effects of illness on your diabetes. You may also need small amounts of drinks containing glucose. If you can't eat, a day or two without food will not matter too much, but drinking plenty of sugar-free fluids throughout the day is essential to prevent dehydration.

Diarrhoea and vomiting

Episodes of sickness and diarrhoea may be short-lived, but they can affect your diabetes within a few hours.

Type 1 diabetes

With type 1 diabetes, If you become hyperglycaemic and dehydrated as a result of prolonged vomiting and

▽ **Aiding recovery**
When you are ill, it is especially important to continue to take your diabetes medication, to check your blood glucose frequently, and to keep hydrated in order to recover as quickly as possible.

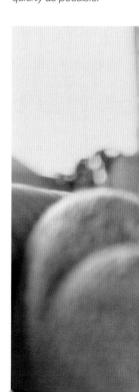

diarrhoea, and are unable to keep any food or fluids down, your body may produce ketones. A large amount of these substances leads to a serious condition known as diabetic ketoacidosis, or DKA (see p.71). You can help to prevent DKA by always taking your insulin, even if you are not eating or are vomiting. However, you need to check your urine or blood for ketones to assess the seriousness of your condition. If your blood or urine does contain ketones, or if you have diarrhoea and vomiting that continues for more than 2–3 hours, contact your health professional urgently.

Type 2 diabetes

With type 2 diabetes, you are at low risk of developing diabetic ketoacidosis if you have diarrhoea and vomiting. However, your blood glucose level can still rise extremely high and you can also become very dehydrated, which

COPING WITH ILLNESS

- Check your blood glucose at least once every 2 hours to learn how the illness is affecting your blood glucose. If you can't do the tests yourself, ask a relative or friend or contact your health professional.

- Continue to take your diabetes medication, even if you are not eating.

- Make sure you keep well hydrated by drinking 2–3 litres of sugar-free fluids throughout the day.

- If you are not able to eat solid food, try milk, fruit juice, or soup at mealtimes.

- If you are vomiting and unable to keep any food or drink down, contact your health professional urgently.

- If you have type 1 diabetes, take small mouthfuls of drinks containing glucose every hour to help prevent ketones from forming.

- If you are ill and are not sure what to do, contact your health professional for advice.

can lead to a condition known as hyperosmolar hyperglycaemic state, or HHS (see p.71). If you are unable to take your diabetes medication or keep any fluids down, contact your health professional immediately.

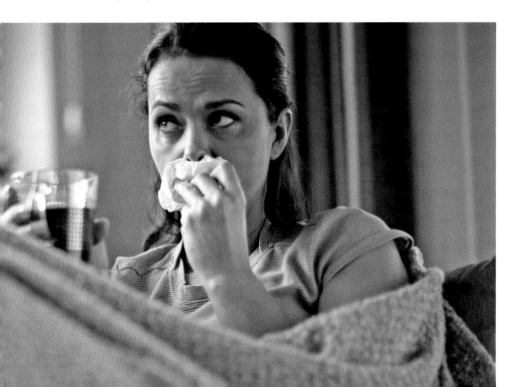

Taking medication

Alongside your diabetes medication, you may need to take other prescribed medication, either short-term for a temporary illness or long-term for an ongoing condition. You may also choose to use over-the-counter medications or take supplements or complementary remedies. You need to be aware of how other medications can affect your diabetes so that you can continue to manage it successfully.

Prescription medications

Short-term treatment with medication prescribed by a doctor or other healthcare professional is frequently all that is needed to treat a wide range of common illnesses. For example, a bacterial infection of the sinuses causing sinusitis often clears up with a short course of antibiotics. In such cases, the antibiotics may also benefit your blood glucose levels, which may have been raised by the infection. Certain prescription medications for ongoing conditions may also affect blood glucose levels or the management of your diabetes. For example, corticosteroid tablets or injections, which may be prescribed to treat inflammatory conditions such as rheumatoid arthritis, cause a rise in blood glucose. Some hormone treatments, such as thyroid hormones to treat an underactive thyroid gland, may also cause a rise in blood glucose. However, the contraceptive pill (see p.118) does not significantly affect blood glucose levels. Beta blockers, which may sometimes be used to treat high blood pressure, may reduce your awareness of the early symptoms of a hypoglycaemic episode (see pp.62–67).

The effects of any prescribed medication on your diabetes depend on the specific drug and also on its form. As a result, if you are prescribed medication it is vital to tell the healthcare professional that you have diabetes and the medication (if any) you use to manage it. In some cases, the healthcare professional may be able to prescribe a medication that has little or no effect on blood glucose or a form of medication that minimizes its effects on blood glucose – for example, taking a medication via skin patches or an inhaler tends to affect blood glucose less than tablets or injections. If an alternative medication or form of

---

USING MEDICATION SAFELY

When you have diabetes, it is important to take special care with medications because of their potential for affecting your diabetes management.

- For any medication, always read the label and the patient information leaflet. If you still have queries about any aspect of the medication, talk to a pharmacist, the prescriber, or other healthcare professional before using it.

- If you are prescribed new medication, make sure you tell the prescriber that you have diabetes and all the medications you are already using, including any non-prescribed medications or remedies.

- If you experience any adverse effects from a medication or remedy that has not been prescribed or recommended by a healthcare professional or if it interferes with your diabetes management, stop using that product.

- If you buy medications online, only use an officially registered online pharmacy to ensure that the medications are of guaranteed quality.

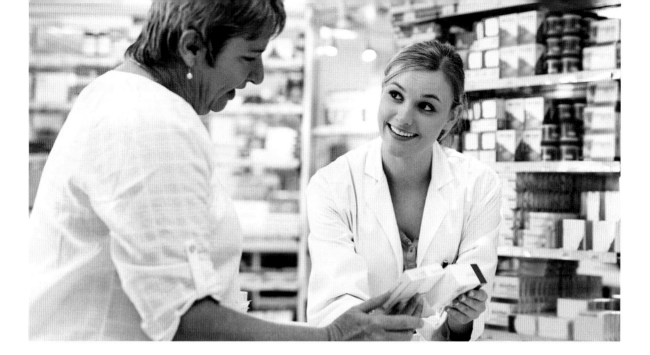

medication is not an option, you should make sure the prescriber gives you detailed information about how your diabetes management can be adjusted. Your diabetes health professional will also be able to give you advice.

Over-the-counter medications

Some medicines that you can buy over the counter may contain sugar, for example, some syrups for coughs and colds, which can interfere with your blood glucose management. If sugar-free or low-sugar formulations are available, these are preferable as they will have less effect on your blood glucose. If you have other conditions in addition to diabetes, some over-the-counter medications may be harmful. For example, if you have peripheral neuropathy (see pp.188–189) or reduced circulation (see peripheral ischaemia, pp.189–190), some treatments for corns, calluses, or fungal infections may damage your feet. In addition, certain over-the-counter medications may have adverse interactions with your diabetes medication or medication you are taking for other conditions. Before using any non-prescription medications, always read the patient information leaflets and obtain specific advice from a pharmacist or other healthcare professional.

Supplements and complementary medications

None of the wide range of dietary supplements and complementary medications available will cure or treat diabetes or substitute for your prescribed diabetes medication. Depending on the specific product, they may have unpredictable effects on your blood glucose or may interact with your diabetes medication and cause side effects. It is wise to get advice from your healthcare professional or a registered alternative therapy practitioner before using such products. If you do decide to use them, try to monitor your blood glucose carefully while you are taking them.

△ **Choosing medication**
Many medications and remedies can be bought without a prescription. Before choosing a product, always check with a pharmacist or other healthcare professional and tell them that you have diabetes.

Going into hospital

If you need to go into hospital – whether or not it is related to your diabetes – it will still be necessary to manage your diabetes carefully. Hospital procedures and schedules (for mealtimes, for example) may be different from those you are used to at home, but being aware of what to expect and preparing for it will help your visit be trouble-free.

Planned inpatient admission

If you know you are going into hospital for an inpatient procedure, you can plan ahead for it with the hospital staff and your diabetes health professionals. A planned admission gives you the chance to discuss how much involvement you will have in your diabetes management and what the hospital staff will provide if you are unable to manage your diabetes yourself as a result of your procedure. You will be able to find out about the timings and types of food that will be provided, to decide whether you will need to bring hypoglycaemia remedies or snacks. You can ask about what diabetes equipment you will need to bring with you, because some items may not be available, such as flash monitor or continuous glucose monitor sensors, although insulin and other diabetes medications are likely to be provided. You can also find out about the diabetes specialist team in the hospital, and ask to talk to them them before you are admitted if you need to.

Emergency admission

If you have to go into hospital because of a medical emergency, you may not have your own equipment available, and you will have less control over how your diabetes is managed. If you are able to, tell the hospital staff about your diabetes and its treatment. However, the staff will look after your diabetes using hospital procedures. For example, if you can't eat, you will be given glucose and insulin via a drip, and you will have frequent blood glucose checks so that the insulin and glucose can be adjusted as needed. When you can eat properly again, your regular or adjusted treatment will restart and the drip will be removed.

> ### PREPARING FOR A HOSPITAL STAY
>
> - Find out if there is a hospital diabetes specialist team and how to contact them before admission to discuss your diabetes management when in hospital.
> - Take your usual diabetes medications and equipment into hospital and/or a complete list of everything you use.
> - If your treatment can cause hypos, inform the hospital staff how you usually treat them.
> - Always carry your diabetes identification (including what type of diabetes you have) in case you have to be admitted to hospital in an emergency.

If you to go into hospital, always tell the healthcare professionals what type of diabetes you have

Outpatient and day-care procedures

As with a planned inpatient admission, for procedures that do not need an overnight hospital stay you will have the chance beforehand to plan how to manage your diabetes in conjunction with the health professionals. For example, if you have to fast before the procedure, you will need advice on extra blood glucose checks and whether you will need to adjust your diabetes medication. When you leave hospital afterwards, you will probably be able to resume managing your diabetes in the usual way, although sometimes you may need to adjust it.

Discharge from hospital

During your hospital stay, changes may have been made to your diabetes treatment. You can discuss any changes with the hospital health professionals before you leave, and you will be able to ask questions or see the diabetes specialist team so that you understand any new regimen or medication. If you have been eating differently from usual or have been less active in hospital than at home, you may be at risk of hypoglycaemia when you resume your usual activities, so you can also find out whether you will need to make further adjustments once you are back at home.

▽ **Intravenous drip**
When in hospital, you may be given glucose and insulin directly into a vein via a drip. When you have recovered and can take medication and eat as usual, the drip will be removed.

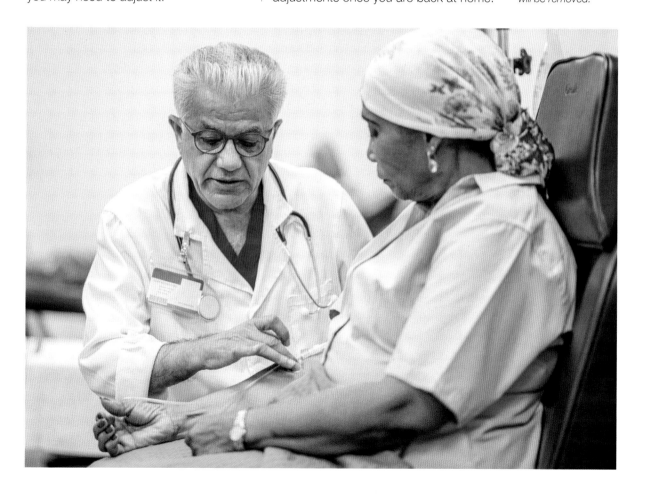

Women's health

If you are a woman with diabetes, it can be useful to know how your hormones and common female experiences can affect your blood glucose level so that you can take steps to look after your health and minimize the effect on your diabetes.

Your menstrual cycle

During your menstrual cycle, levels of oestrogen and progesterone rise and fall. At the start of your cycle, oestrogen causes the lining of the uterus to thicken. This is then maintained by rising progesterone levels during the second half of your cycle. If conception does not occur, progesterone levels fall, triggering shedding of the lining of the uterus. These hormonal changes may affect blood glucose levels. If you think this might be happening to you, recording your blood glucose four or more times a day just before, during, and directly after your period will help you to identify any pattern.

If your blood glucose tends to rise just before your period, you could:

● Try fitting in some extra physical activity to bring your blood glucose level down.

● Try to limit extra or sugar-rich food.

● Try increasing your dose of insulin or other medication in the few days before your period is due.

If, on the other hand, your blood glucose is lower than normal and you have a tendency to have more hypos, you could:

● Try increasing your intake of carbohydrate-containing foods.

● Reduce your insulin or medication dose in the few days before your period.

The way in which your periods affect your blood glucose is individual but likely to remain fairly constant, so even if you change your diabetes treatment, over time you should be able to work out how to keep your blood glucose balanced throughout your monthly cycle.

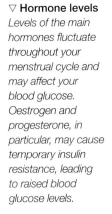

▽ **Hormone levels**
Levels of the main hormones fluctuate throughout your menstrual cycle and may affect your blood glucose. Oestrogen and progesterone, in particular, may cause temporary insulin resistance, leading to raised blood glucose levels.

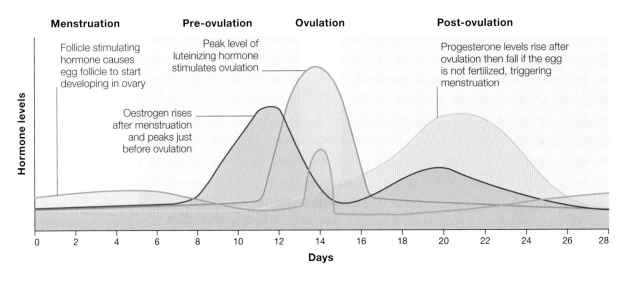

Menstruation

Follicle stimulating hormone causes egg follicle to start developing in ovary

Oestrogen rises after menstruation and peaks just before ovulation

Pre-ovulation

Peak level of luteinizing hormone stimulates ovulation

Ovulation

Post-ovulation

Progesterone levels rise after ovulation then fall if the egg is not fertilized, triggering menstruation

Hormone levels

0   2   4   6   8   10   12   14   16   18   20   22   24   26   28

Days

Menopause

Many changes occur in a woman's body during the menopause, but these will not necessarily affect your diabetes and its treatment. However, you may find that some symptoms of the menopause are similar to those that occur when you have a high or low blood glucose level. If you do feel hot, shaky, or start sweating, taking a blood glucose reading can help you decide whether you need to treat your diabetes at this time. You may wish to consider hormone replacement therapy (HRT), which may help to relieve menopausal symptoms. Ask your health professional whether taking HRT would be right for you.

Changes in levels of hormones during your menstrual cycle may affect blood glucose levels

Stress, emotions, and hormone levels

Mood swings and feeling emotional at times of hormonal change, such as periods and the menopause, are common but are usually short-lived. However, managing diabetes can cause extra stress (see pp.110–111). If your low mood or emotional changes are becoming persistent, extra support and treatment may help (see pp.176–179).

MENOPAUSE SYMPTOMS AND DIABETES

Some menopause symptoms can mimic hypoglycaemia (see pp.64–65) or hyperglycaemia (see pp.70–71). The only way to tell what the symptoms are due to is check your blood glucose level.

MENOPAUSE SYMPTOMS	SIMILAR DIABETES-RELATED SYMPTOMS
Hot flushes and night sweats	Hypos may cause sweating
Palpitations	Palpitations and a fast pulse may be signs of a hypo
Mood changes, such as low mood	Hypos can cause a change in mood
Headaches	Hyperglycaemia may cause headaches due to dehydration. A hypo in the night may cause a headache on waking
Difficulty sleeping, causing tiredness and irritabity during the day	Hypos can cause tiredness. Being irritable or anxious may also be signs of a hypo. Hyperglycaemia may mean you get up at night frequently to go to the toilet, resulting in tiredness during the day
Problems with memory and concentration	Problems with concentration may result from hyperglycaemia or hypoglycaemia
Recurrent urinary tract infections	Hyperglycaemia may cause urinary tract infections
Vaginal dryness, and pain, itching, or discomfort during sex; reduced libido	Hyperglycaemia can cause thrush (candidiasis), producing vaginal itching
Joint stiffness, aches and pains, and reduced muscle mass	Hyperglycaemia may cause muscle cramps

Pregnancy

It is important to plan your pregnancy carefully so that your blood glucose is well-managed before you conceive. Throughout your pregnancy, looking after your diabetes and attending antenatal appointments will mean you and your baby are as healthy as possible.

Planning for pregnancy

Before you stop contraception, your diabetes health professional will work with you to make sure both your general health and diabetes management are the best they can be, to help ensure a healthy pregnancy. This means that you will need to take high-dose folic acid supplements, and take extra care over your blood glucose levels.

You should be checking your blood glucose at least 4 times a day and make sure that most of your levels are in the range of 4–7 millimoles per litre (mmol/L). You may need to work towards this by adjusting your insulin, tablets, food intake, and activity level. If this is difficult or causes lots of hypos, you may need to change your insulin regimen – for example, from twice-daily injections to a mutidose injection regimen (see pp.46–51) – or consider using a pump (see p.54). These enable you to match your dose to your glucose level more closely.

If you take tablets for your diabetes, you may need to have insulin injections instead to achieve the blood glucose levels you need before becoming pregnant. When you do conceive, you will probably need to switch to insulin. Your health professional will also review any other medications you take – for example, to treat raised blood pressure or cholesterol – as some cannot be taken during pregnancy.

When you are pregnant

Intensive blood-glucose management is crucial while you are pregnant, both for your baby's and your own health. If your blood glucose is raised, your baby's will be, too. This is because glucose can cross your placenta into your baby's blood but insulin cannot. If your baby's glucose is high, they will have to produce more insulin to lower it, which causes extra glucose to be stored in your baby's body, resulting in faster growth. Keeping your blood glucose in your target range during pregnancy is also important to prevent ketones from forming (see p.71). These can be very harmful to your baby. They may form even if your blood glucose is not

---

DEALING WITH HYPOS DURING PREGNANCY

- If you are using insulin, be alert for extra hypos during the first 3 months, due to increased sensitivity to insulin, especially combined with eating less if you have morning sickness.

- Eat starchy carbohydrates regularly throughout the day to reduce the likelihood of having a hypo.

- Check your blood glucose level at least 4 times a day and adjust your insulin according to the results.

- Keep glucose tablets, a glucose drink, or dextrose gel with you at all times to use as soon as you feel hypo symptoms coming on.

- Tell your partner, a friend, or a work colleague that hypoglycaemia could occur and, if possible, show them how to give you a glucagon injection (see p.67) if you become unconscious.

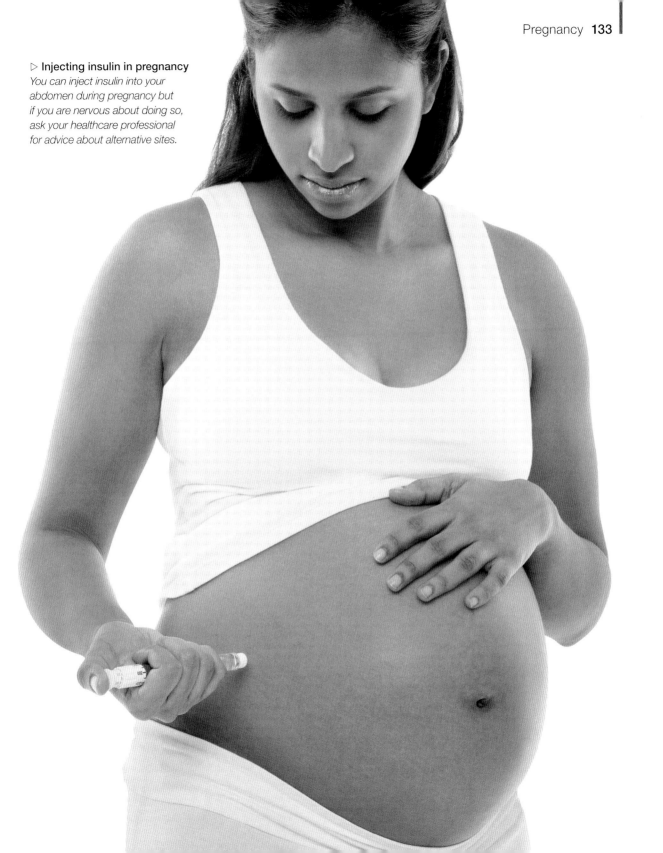

▷ **Injecting insulin in pregnancy**
You can inject insulin into your abdomen during pregnancy but if you are nervous about doing so, ask your healthcare professional for advice about alternative sites.

high enough to give you symptoms, so it is vital that you increase your insulin dose as soon as your blood glucose starts to rise.

You need to monitor your blood glucose levels frequently and make sure you keep your blood glucose level well within target range:

- 4–5.3 mmol/L on waking.
- 4–7.8 mmol/L one hour after a meal.
- 4–6.4 mmol/L two hours after a meal.

Your health professional will also give you an HbA1c test (see p.31); ideally, your HbA1c level should be 48 mmol/mol (6.5 per cent) during pregnancy. As your pregnancy progresses, you will need larger doses of insulin to keep your blood glucose at these levels.

If you have type 1 diabetes, you may be offered a continuous glucose monitoring system (see p.33 and p.35)

ANTENATAL TESTS*

You will have several antenatal tests at intervals throughout your pregnancy, starting as soon as your pregnancy is confirmed. In addition to the standard tests offered to every pregnant woman, certain specific tests are needed when you have diabetes. Some tests may be repeated more often than indicated if there are concerns.

	PROCEDURE	WHEN	REASON
TESTS FOR WOMEN WITH DIABETES	Blood sample for HbA1c	At start of pregnancy (unless recently checked); every 3 months during pregnancy.	To check that your blood glucose level is within recommended range, to ensure your baby can grow and develop healthily, and to help prevent pregnancy problems (see opposite).
	Retinal (eye) examination	Start of pregnancy (unless recently checked) and at 28 weeks; more often if you already have or develop retinopathy.	To look for signs of retinopathy (see pp.180–181), which can develop or worsen during pregnancy.
	Blood sample for kidney function	At start of pregnancy (unless recently checked); during pregnancy if you already have or develop kidney problems.	To ensure that your kidneys are functioning well.
ROUTINE TESTS FOR ALL PREGNANT WOMEN	Urine sample	At every visit (every 1–2 weeks when you have diabetes).	To check for the presence of protein, which can indicate pre-eclampsia (see opposite); also to detect infection or ketones.
	Blood sample for anaemia, blood group, and rhesus D factor	At start of pregnancy (unless taken during pre-pregnancy planning).	To ensure healthy iron levels; to check your blood group in case you need a blood transfusion and also so that you can be offered anti-D treatment if needed.
	Ultrasound scan	At approximately 12 and 20 weeks. Additional scans for women with diabetes at 28, 32, and 36 weeks.	To assess the development and growth of your baby, including checks for specific problems, such as spina bifida, and a specialist heart scan.
	Blood pressure	At every visit.	To check for raised blood pressure, which increases the risk of pre-eclampsia (see opposite).
	Fetal wellbeing monitoring	At every visit, usually by the midwife or consultant, but sometimes also using a cardiotocograph (fetal heart monitor).	To check your baby's size, heartbeat, and movements. You will also be asked to keep a daily chart of your baby's movements at home.

to use during pregnancy. This can make the intensive monitoring of your blood glucose levels easier.

Physical and mental wellbeing

Having diabetes and being pregnant is hard work. You have to cope with lots of appointments and probably pay more attention than usual to your diabetes care. It's as important to look after your mental health as well as all the physical aspects of being pregnant. Finding someone to listen to your worries, share in planning, attend appointments with you, and encourage you to keep going with your diabetes care can be very helpful. Techniques such as yoga or deep breathing every day help you relax. Eating extra-healthily, being physically active on a regular basis – a brisk daily walk or swimming – will all increase your chances of a successful pregnancy.

Planning the birth

You may need special care during labour, so you will be advised to have your baby in hospital. Your health professional will discuss the options available to you and what you can expect to happen to you and your baby during the birth. To help avoid any problems in late pregnancy, you will be advised to give birth between 37 and 39 weeks of pregnancy, by labour being induced or by caesarean section. In some situations, such as if you have any diabetes or pregnancy complications, you may be offered a caesarean section or induction of labour before 37 weeks.

POTENTIAL PREGNANCY PROBLEMS

Most pregnancies progress smoothly, but all pregnant women face potential problems. Having diabetes makes some problems more likely, but the risks can be reduced by healthy eating, regular physical activity, intensive blood glucose monitoring, and careful management of your blood glucose levels.

PROBLEM	IMPLICATIONS
Worsening of diabetes complications	Eye complications, such as retinopathy, may worsen in pregnancy, so your eyes are checked as part of your antenatal care. Kidney problems before pregnancy can increase your risk of raised blood pressure, so this is also checked regularly.
Baby larger than usual	A raised blood glucose level can cause your baby to grow at an increased rate. Keeping your blood glucose levels in their target range reduces this risk. If your baby is larger than usual, they may need to be delivered early.
Polyhydramnios (excessive amniotic fluid)	If your baby has a raised blood glucose level, they may produce more urine. This can lead to an excessive amount of amniotic fluid in the uterus (a condition known as polyhydramnios), which can cause premature labour.
Pre-eclampsia (high blood pressure and protein in the urine)	You will be monitored carefully for pre-eclampsia during clinic visits to detect it early and avoid it leading to eclampsia, which causes seizures and may bring on a coma. If you have high blood pressure, protein in your urine, and fluid retention in the last 3 months of pregnancy, you will be monitored in hospital until your baby is born, and your labour may be induced.
Premature labour	If labour starts before the 37th week of pregnancy, or you are induced early, your baby's lungs may not be fully mature and your baby may need special care when born.

Gestational diabetes

Some women develop diabetes for the first time during pregnancy – this is gestational diabetes. It may be permanent but usually disappears once your baby is born. Even if it disappears, you still have a high risk of developing type 2 diabetes in the near future, which you can take steps to prevent.

Diagnosis

If you have risk factors, such as previous gestational diabetes or a family history of diabetes, your blood glucose will be checked at your first antenatal visit. If not, it will be checked at around 24–28 weeks of pregnancy. If you are diagnosed with gestational diabetes, you will be offered more frequent clinic appointments and support from health professionals.

Treatment and monitoring

Your initial treatment may involve adjusting your food. Limiting food and drinks that are high in sugar and not eating too much carbohydrate can make a big difference to your blood glucose. Your health professional will show you how to check your blood glucose (see pp.36–37) to see how effective changes to your eating habits have been. The ideal blood glucose targets are to have all readings above 4 millimoles per litre (mmol/L), and up to 5.3 mmol/L on waking, 7.8 mmol/L 1 hour after a meal, and 6.4 mmol/L 2 hours after a meal. You will also be given an HbA1c test (see p.31). In pregnancy, the healthy HbA1c level is 48 mmol/mol (6.5 per cent).

If healthier eating is not enough to keep your blood glucose level in the recommended range, you will be offered regular insulin injections or one of the few tablets that are safe to use in pregnancy.

Birth and postnatal care

There is a chance that your baby will need to be delivered by caesarean section or need care in a special unit, so you will be advised to have your baby in hospital. During labour, you may need a glucose drip and insulin infusion and more frequent monitoring (see p.138).

As soon as your baby is born, your need for insulin will reduce dramatically. You may no longer require insulin or need to check your blood glucose. But because there is a risk of developing permanent diabetes when you are pregnant, about 6 weeks after the birth (or sooner if you have symptoms) you will have a fasting blood glucose and HbA1c test, and sometimes also an oral glucose tolerance test (see p.21).

Future diabetes risk

Once you have had temporary gestational diabetes, it is likely to recur in future pregnancies. You are also much more likely to develop type 2 diabetes within a few years. You can help to prevent or delay this by breastfeeding, regular activity, eating healthily, and keeping a healthy weight. There are prevention programmes to support you with this. You will also be offered a blood test every year to check for diabetes and advised to see a health professional if you develop symptoms.

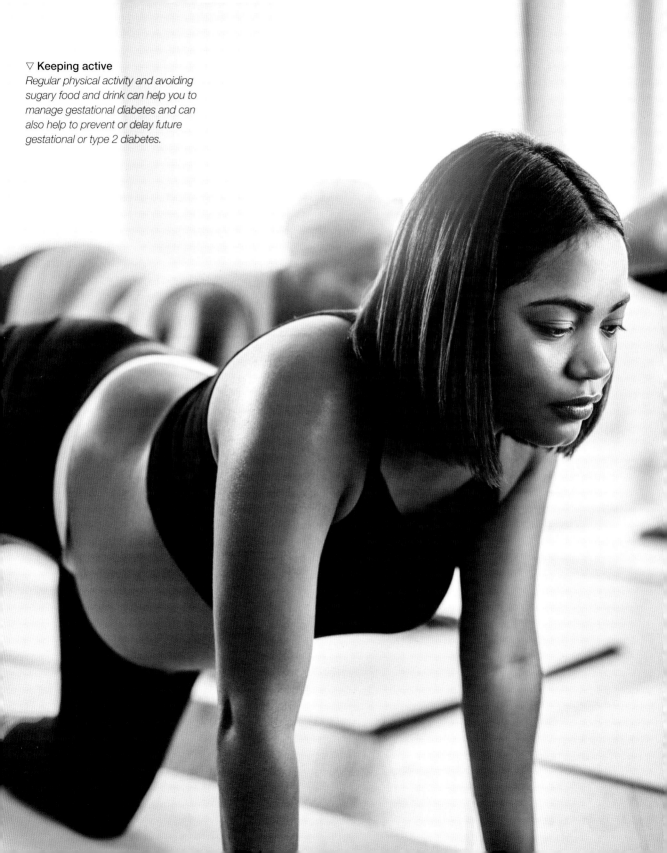

▽ **Keeping active**
Regular physical activity and avoiding sugary food and drink can help you to manage gestational diabetes and can also help to prevent or delay future gestational or type 2 diabetes.

Giving birth

For many women with type 1 or type 2 diabetes, giving birth is similar to any other woman's experience, in most respects, especially if your pregnancy has been problem-free. However, your blood glucose will be closely monitored throughout labour and delivery, and you may need intravenous glucose and insulin. Straight after the birth, your baby's glucose levels will be checked, too.

Labour and blood glucose levels

Your labour may start naturally before 37 weeks. In this case, contact your hospital for advice; also check your blood glucose at least once an hour, or ask somebody else to do it for you, if that is easier. Taking regular blood glucose readings will tell you how the onset of labour is affecting you and will help hospital staff to support you. After 37 weeks, you will be advised to have labour induced or to have a caesarean section.

If you have type 1 diabetes, if labour lasts a long time, or if it starts when your glucose level may be falling (for example, when you have not eaten for some time), you will be offered an intravenous glucose drip to keep your blood glucose stable until the birth. You will also be given an intravenous infusion of insulin. The amounts of glucose and insulin will be adjusted according to your blood glucose level.

Monitoring and pain relief

Your baby's heart rate, position, and movements will be checked throughout your labour. You can have the same pain relief as any other mother who does not have diabetes, depending on how your labour is progressing.

After your baby is born

Once your baby is separated from your placenta, their blood glucose level may fall. For this reason, when your baby is born, a blood sample will be taken to check whether they are hypoglycaemic. In some specific circumstances, such as premature birth, your baby's lungs may not be fully developed. As a result, their breathing will also be checked and, if necessary, they will be helped to breathe at first.

If you and your baby are well after the birth, you will be encouraged to feed your baby immediately. However, if your baby's glucose level is low, they may also need a glucose injection or a tube feed. If your baby is seriously hypoglycaemic or is having difficulty breathing, they may be moved to a special care baby unit.

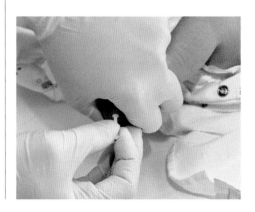

◁ **Blood test**
Your baby will have a heel prick test a couple of hours after birth to check their blood glucose level. If it is low, they will have further tests until it rises; if their blood glucose remains very low, your baby may be transferred to a special care unit.

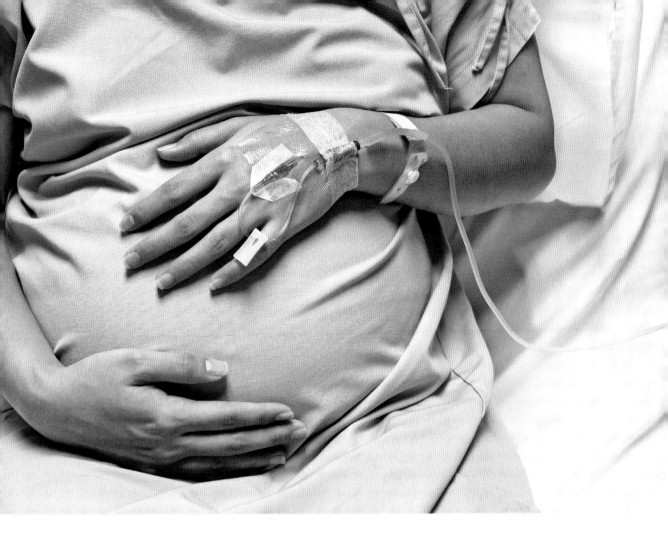

After delivery of your placenta, your need for insulin falls quickly. If you were receiving an insulin infusion during labour, the dose will be lowered or stopped immediately to prevent hypoglycaemia.

Managing your diabetes after the birth
Unless you had a general anaesthetic, you will be able to eat and drink soon after the birth. You should then be able to take over managing your glucose testing and insulin injections if you have them.

If you were on tablets before you were pregnant, you may need to keep taking insulin until you wean your baby. You can't take most tablets for diabetes while you are breastfeeding, because they will affect your baby via your milk.

If you weren't taking insulin or tablets before your pregnancy, you may be able to resume or start blood glucose management through healthy eating and physical activity, in which case there are no special issues about breastfeeding.

△ **Intravenous treatment**
If you have type 1 diabetes, your labour is prolonged, or your blood glucose level falls, you will need intravenous glucose and insulin to keep your blood glucose level stable.

When your **baby is born**, a blood sample will be taken to **check** whether they are **hypoglycaemic**

Life with a new baby

Meals, sleep, and time to yourself or with your partner are all likely to be disrupted once your baby is born, and your diabetes routine is also likely to be upset. Although you can be a little less strict about your blood glucose than when you were pregnant, you still need to aim for a healthy level.

Eating and drinking

It is likely that your usual mealtimes will be disturbed or irregular for a while after having a baby. This can affect how you manage your diabetes and disrupt your blood glucose levels. If you go without food for too long and you take insulin or insulin-stimulating tablets, you may become hypoglycaemic or, if there are long periods of time between your insulin doses, your blood glucose level may rise.

One way to deal with this is to eat regularly, even though it may sometimes be difficult to have a main meal. You may find it useful to prepare or set aside food such as fruit, sandwiches, or cereal bars each day in case you are unable to eat or drink when planned. If your mealtimes are unpredictable and you take a ready-mixed insulin or are on a twice-a-day regimen, changing to a more flexible multidose regimen might suit your new lifestyle better (see pp.46–47).

Breastfeeding

When you breastfeed, you transfer energy to your baby through your milk. This means that you will need to eat additional carbohydrate each day to compensate for the energy you are giving your baby. Like other new mothers who are breastfeeding, you will probably find that you need to drink more sugar-free fluid than normal to prevent yourself from becoming dehydrated.

If you take insulin or insulin-stimulating medication, you may also need to reduce your dose in order to prevent hypoglycaemia. Keep your hypo treatments (such as glucose tablets or glucose drinks) and snacks to hand whenever you are breastfeeding.

Try not to put your baby's feeds before your own food needs. If you feel a hypo coming on, treat it straight away, whether or not you can check your blood glucose level.

 HOW TO RELIEVE STRESS

- Try fitting in some physical activity whenever you can – even just going for a walk outside can help.

- Meet other new parents and share your experiences. There are usually local support groups, including for parents with diabetes.

- Ask for support from family and friends – they might be able to give practical help and/or emotional support.

- Rest and sleep whenever you can. Ongoing tiredness can contribute to stress and low mood, and sleep can improve them.

Sleeping

If you sleep when your baby sleeps, you will probably be napping throughout the day. This could result in a hypo if you doze when you are due to eat a meal, or hyperglycaemia if you sleep in and miss your injection time because you were awake most of the night. If necessary, have a snack when you get up to feed your baby at night.

You may need to consider how to adapt your insulin regimen if your sleeping pattern is unpredictable and is causing troublesome swings in your blood glucose.

Stress and mood

Looking after your new baby and trying to manage your diabetes can be very stressful. After working so hard to manage your blood glucose during pregnancy, it can be difficult to relax this and return to your pre-pregnancy target levels. Finding time to check your blood glucose, eat, and take medication as you would like may also be a strain.

It is not unusual for new mothers to feel slightly low in mood during the first few days or weeks after childbirth. Having diabetes won't make you any more or less likely to experience this mood change, sometimes known as the "baby blues", nor more serious postnatal depression. However, feeling like this can affect your energy levels and your ability to manage your diabetes as well as your new baby's needs. If you feel you are not coping, talking to your health professional about how you feel is important so that they can help you, perhaps, for example, with a mood assessment and practical suggestions for coping strategies. If you experience ongoing depression, you may need treatment (see pp.176–179).

Letting your **family and friends** help can **ease** the **stress** of dealing with a **new baby** and managing your **diabetes**

If you are already having treatment for a pre-existing mental health or emotional problem, or another health condition in addition to your diabetes, these need to be reassessed. It may be necessary for your diabetes and/or other treatment to be adjusted.

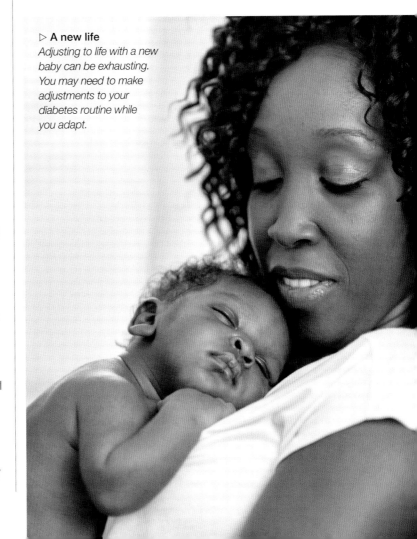

▷ **A new life**
Adjusting to life with a new baby can be exhausting. You may need to make adjustments to your diabetes routine while you adapt.

Benefiting from health care*

When you have diabetes, regular health checks are an integral part of life, with several routine appointments a year, plus extra ones if required, and an annual review. You and your healthcare professionals are partners in your care, and these consultations provide an opportunity to review your diabetes management and health, and also to keep you informed about new developments.

Routine appointments

You will be invited for several routine appointments every year with your diabetes health professionals, typically three or four but sometimes more. You may also request additional consultations if you feel you need them.

A routine appointment usually includes measurements of your blood glucose and HbA1c levels (see p.31) and other medical checks in the care plan from your annual review. Your weight will also be measured, if necessary. Otherwise, the appointments are focused on how you are managing your life with diabetes and any problems you may be having. The appointments can not only help you to manage your diabetes, they also provide an opportunity to ask questions, build a relationship with your health professional, and broaden your knowledge – perhaps by finding out about new pieces of equipment, diabetes support groups, or research projects.

Annual review

Once a year you will be invited to attend an annual review with your diabetes health professionals. This is your main overall diabetes health check, and it covers the physical, psychological, and educational aspects of the condition. Your health professionals will check your health, offer treatment, and make any necessary referrals to other specialists.

◁ **Obtaining a blood sample**
As part of your regular checks, you will have blood taken from a vein in your arm, in order to get a large enough sample for several different tests. This may happen before or during your appointment.

↘ **KEEPING UP TO DATE**

Being well-informed about new developments helps you take an active part in the care you are offered. Some ways you can do this are:

- Signing up for online updates from national diabetes associations.
- Making contact with other people living with diabetes for peer support.
- Regularly checking for news and updates from the manufacturers of your insulin, medication, and diabetes equipment.

ANNUAL REVIEW MEDICAL CHECKS

 Blood tests to measure levels of lipids (cholesterol and fats), glucose, and HbA1c (see p.31).

 Blood and urine tests to check the functioning of your kidneys.

 Blood pressure measurement, as part of the assessment of your heart and circulation.

 Height and weight measurement to calculate your body mass index, and waist measurement (see pp.92–93).

 Examining your feet and legs to assess blood circulation and nerve function, as checks for early signs of peripheral ischaemia or peripheral neuropathy (see pp.188–190).

 Imaging of the retina at the back of your eyes to check for any changes that may indicate retinopathy (see pp.180–181).

 If you use injected medication, checking your injection sites for build-up of fatty deposits in your skin (see lipohypertrophy, p.198).

They will also help you with any concerns you may have about any aspect of your diabetes, and it can be useful if you prepare for your review by making a list of these beforehand. If you have the results of recent blood tests or any other health checks, the annual review provides an opportunity to discuss the results with your diabetes healthcare professionals.

Your annual review may take place in a single session or over several sessions. In addition to medical checks, your health professional will ask about your general health, such as whether you smoke, drink alcohol, and if you have any diabetes-related health issues, such as urinary problems (see pp.184–187) or sexual dysfunction (see p.201). Your review will also include discussions about how you feel you are managing your life with diabetes, such as:

- Whether you feel distressed, burnt out, or depressed by diabetes (see pp.110–111 and pp.176–179) and if you need psychological support.
- How you are coping with food and eating and how to obtain individual support from a specialist dietitian.
- Whether you are planning to become pregnant and, if so, how to prepare for it.

As a result of your annual review, you and your health professional will decide on a care plan for your diabetes, including any agreed changes to your existing regimen, any new medication, further appointments, any medical checks for your routine appointments, and contact details of who you can ask for advice or support. You may also be invited to attend a diabetes education session or event. You and your health professional will have a written copy of the plan, so everything is documented.

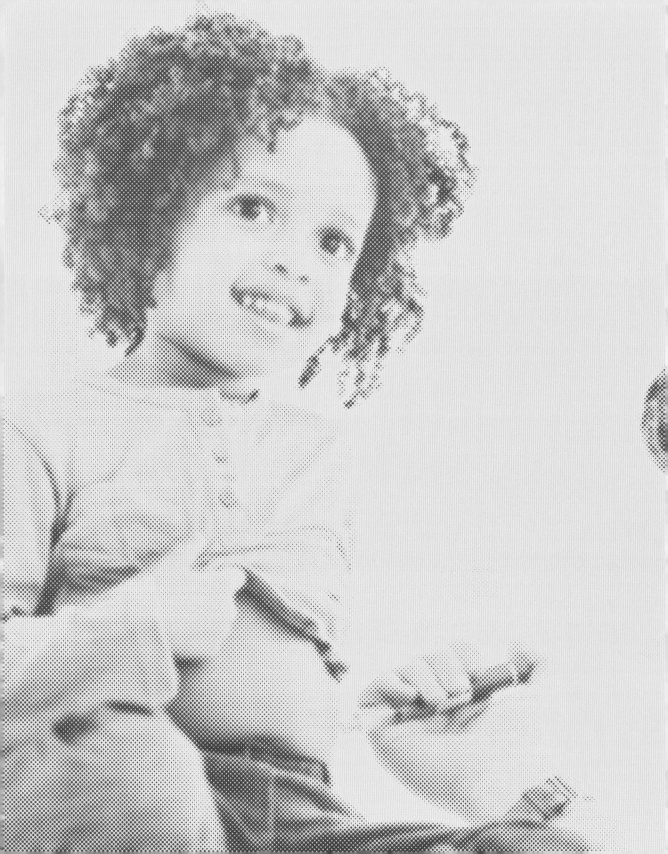

Children and young people

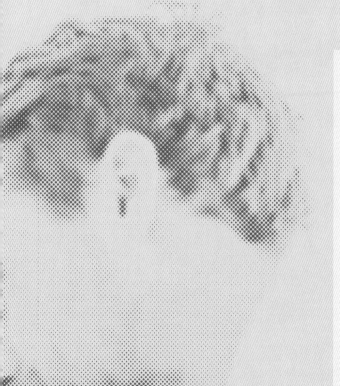

Babies and young children

Caring for a baby or young child with diabetes places many demands on you as a parent. You need to manage their insulin, blood glucose, and healthy eating, as well as deal with hypos. Getting support and learning how to deal with the emotional impact of diabetes will help.

Your child's diagnosis

It is rare for children under five to develop diabetes, but type 1 diabetes can occur in babies and toddlers from the age of about one year onwards. The symptoms, such as passing a lot of urine and being very thirsty, are the same in children under five as in adults (see pp.18–19). They can become apparent very quickly – over just a few days or a week. Once your child has been diagnosed with diabetes, you will be offered support, advice, and routine check-ups from your health professional and diabetes team.

Learning about diabetes and emotional impact

When your baby or young child is first diagnosed with diabetes, you are likely to experience various emotions – anger, guilt, anxiety, and sadness, for example. You may worry whether you will be able to cope with the level of care your child will need every day. You will be responsible for looking after all aspects of their diabetes care, which can make your job as a parent even more demanding. Your child needs food at regular intervals, blood checks, and insulin injections. They might not yet be able to tell you how they feel, so it is also your job to make sure that their blood glucose does not fall to a level at which they have a hypo (see pp.62–65 and pp.154–155).

However, you are not alone. With the support of diabetes professionals, you will quickly learn more about diabetes and what you need to do to take care of your child. As well as routine appointments at a diabetes clinic, diabetes health professionals will visit you to discuss your child's growth and development. They will also help you aim for blood glucose levels within certain target ranges (see pp.150–151) so as to keep your child healthy as they grow older.

INFORMING YOUR CHILD'S CARERS

You need to make sure that anyone who looks after your child is given enough information about your child's diabetes. You can ask your health professional to help you provide this.

- Explain what diabetes means, and specifically what treatments and blood glucose checks your child needs and when.

- If carers need to give injections or check your child's blood glucose, show them exactly what is involved. You may need to repeat the information before it becomes familiar.

- Tell carers about your child's eating and drinking requirements (see pp.148–149) and why these are important.

- Explain what symptoms might suggest your child is having a hypo (see pp.62–65), and what they need to do to treat one (see pp.154–155).

- Explain the symptoms of hyperglycaemia (see pp.68–69).

- Tell carers what they should do if your child is unwell, in particular, if your child is vomiting.

Talking to friends and family

Your family and friends will probably be concerned about your child's diabetes, and they will almost certainly want to know more about it. It's up to you to decide how much to say and to whom, but you will need to give more detailed information to people who care for your child, such as school staff, babysitters, or childminders (see opposite). You will find they respond in a variety of ways.

People who are close to you may be upset and unsure how to treat your child. You may find it difficult to support and reassure others when it is all new to you too, but it is important to try to

Try to help people to understand what you are going through, and appreciate how they are feeling, too

help people understand what you are going through and to appreciate how they are feeling too. If you have other children, make sure they are included and don't feel left out. You may need to spend time with them to answer any questions they have about diabetes and any worries they have about their brother or sister.

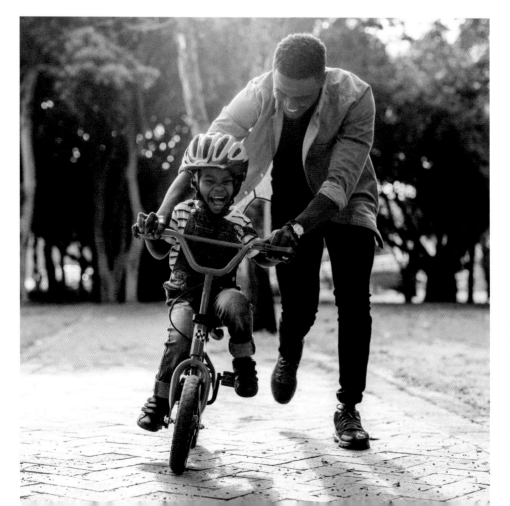

◁ **Happy times**
Having a young child with diabetes is likely to put extra pressure on your role as a parent, but you can still enjoy lots of different activities together despite its demands.

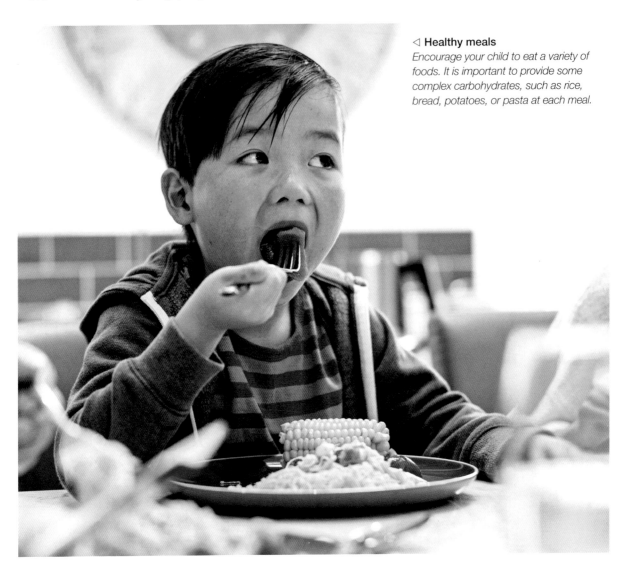

◁ **Healthy meals**
Encourage your child to eat a variety of foods. It is important to provide some complex carbohydrates, such as rice, bread, potatoes, or pasta at each meal.

Babies and young children:
Eating and drinking

Introducing regular food and mealtime routines for your young child will help with their diabetes. As babies move from milk to solids, you can start to introduce a variety of foods, especially carbohydrates, needed to balance blood glucose and avoid hypos (see pp.154–155).

SUPERVISING YOUR CHILD'S FOOD INTAKE

- Mealtimes are important for social as well as for nutritional reasons – avoid them being a source of conflict about food.

- Don't worry if your child doesn't eat healthy food at every meal – it's the overall balance that matters.

- If you're having problems, talk with your health professional about ways of matching your child's insulin to their current eating pattern.

Introducing different foods and drink

Your young child needs a variety of foods to ensure that they grow and develop healthily. If you are breastfeeding, feeding on demand will help to fulfil your baby's nutritional needs, although you may need to supplement breast milk with bottle feeding if your baby's blood glucose becomes low. If low or high blood glucose is a constant problem, adjusting your baby's insulin dose will be helpful.

As you introduce your child to more foods, you will need to include those that contain complex carbohydrates, such as bread, pasta, rice, noodles, and potatoes. Your child will need to eat enough carbohydrate at mealtimes and throughout the day to keep their blood glucose level as close as possible to their target range (see pp.150–151). Snacks could include, for example, yoghurt, milkshakes, cereal bars, or fruit.

You won't do your child any harm if some meals are less healthy than others. As with all children, it is the overall content of their food intake that matters.

Food refusal and dislikes

Your child may be choosy about food at times, and their eating pattern may vary a lot. This can be frustrating when you want to encourage your child to eat in order to keep their blood glucose in the recommended range. If your child refuses food, keep calm. Have an alternative prepared – perhaps one of your child's favourite snack or meals – that will tempt them to eat. Be careful not to offer more than one or two choices though: any more and mealtimes could become a battle of wills between you and your child.

Ensure your child has regular carbohydrate-rich foods to keep blood glucose in the target range

Bedtime snacks

Make sure that your child has eaten enough food in the evening to prevent their blood glucose falling overnight, especially if they usually sleep through until morning. If you don't think your child has eaten enough, and you can't fit in a snack for them before bedtime, you may need to check their blood glucose later in the evening. If it is too low, give your child a drink or snack that's quick and easy to eat. If low or raised blood glucose becomes a regular event, you will need to reduce or increase your child's insulin dose earlier. As your child grows older, and the time between their evening meal and bedtime gets longer, it becomes easier to assess what they will need during the night.

Eating out

There is no reason why you shouldn't eat out as a family when your child has diabetes, whether at a restaurant or a friend's house. Fast food, takeaways, and party food are all good sources of carbohydrate as well as being enjoyable treats on these occasions.

If you are not sure what food will be on offer or when, it can be useful to pack an emergency supply of foods you know your child will eat. In addition, include glucose or another fast-acting carbohydrate source for immediate treatment of a hypo, and longer-acting carbohydrate-containing food to maintain the raised blood glucose afterwards.

Babies and young children:
Blood glucose management

Taking good care of your child's blood glucose is essential right from the start: what you do now could make a difference to their future health as an adult and reduce the risk of long-term complications. Blood glucose management is also important for their healthy growth, development, and wellbeing.

Target blood glucose levels

Blood glucose management for young children is the same as for anybody else with diabetes: the target is blood glucose levels of 4–7 millimoles per litres (mmol/L) before meals, 5–9 mmol/L after, and for HbA1c levels of 48 or below (see p.31). You won't always be able to achieve these exactly, but by keeping records of your child's levels, you can identify patterns and work out what to do about them.

Checking your child's blood glucose level and giving insulin may be hard for you, especially at first. However, to manage your child's diabetes as effectively as possible, you will need to monitor their blood glucose regularly before and/or after meals and at least five times a day (if you use the fingerprick method). The benefit of this is that you can adjust your child's diabetes treatment, activity, or food intake according to the outcomes.

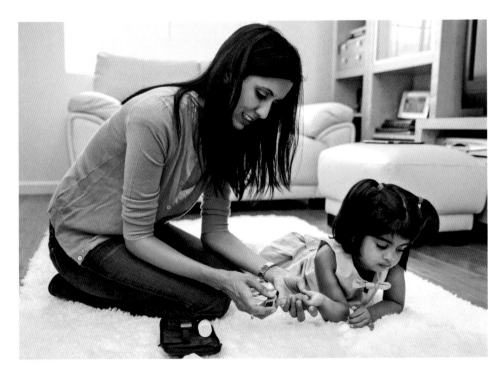

▷ **Checking your child's blood glucose**
When checking your child's blood glucose it is helpful to stay relaxed, do the check as efficiently as possible, and then resume what you were both doing beforehand.

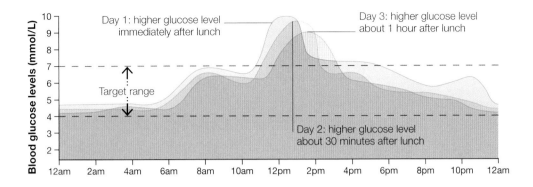

Day 1: higher glucose level immediately after lunch

Day 3: higher glucose level about 1 hour after lunch

Target range

Day 2: higher glucose level about 30 minutes after lunch

Identifying patterns

Any changes you make to your child's diabetes medication, activity, or food intake are best based on a pattern of blood glucose results rather than a single one. For example, higher blood glucose levels occurring at the same time on several consecutive days is a pattern, so you can try to find a cause and take the appropriate action. If there isn't an obvious reason for higher or lower levels, your child may need an adjustment to their insulin dose (see pp.48–51). Continuing to check their blood glucose will show you how well a change has worked.

If your child has a raised blood glucose level, try to avoid allowing this to continue for more than a few days (even if they seem well), because this could increase the chance of your child developing symptoms (see pp.68–69), becoming prone to infection, or starting to produce ketones (see p.71).

Blood glucose management also entails keeping your child's blood glucose level above 4 mmol/L in order to avoid hypos. However, if your child does have a hypo, you should take immediate action (see pp.154–155).

As your child grows older, bigger, and takes part in new activities, you will probably need to adjust how their

△ **Blood glucose patterns**
The pattern of your child's blood glucose levels over several days can help you to identify recurring highs or lows and take appropriate action. For example, if it tends to rise after lunch, that may indicate that you should review their morning activity, food, or insulin dose.

diabetes is managed; they may need a different type of insulin or insulin regimen (see pp.44–47), or adjustments to their food, or both. Your diabetes health professional will be able to give advice that is tailored to support you and your child's needs.

Blood glucose **management** for **young children** is the **same** as for **anybody else** with diabetes

MANAGING YOUR CHILD'S BLOOD GLUCOSE

- Use trends and patterns in your child's blood glucose levels to guide you rather than responding to each individual reading. However, a very low reading – a hypo – does require immediate action.

- Link up with other families with children who have diabetes online or in person for emotional and practical support.

- Keep up to date with new technology that can help you in managing your child's diabetes, such as flash monitors and special insulin pens for children.

- Use appointments with your diabetes health professional to ask questions, discuss worries, and find out the latest information.

Babies and young children:
Blood glucose and insulin

Although you might find it difficult to inject your baby or young child every day, they need insulin to live, and blood glucose checks will always be part of their everyday life. Keeping blood glucose levels in the recommended range is essential from whenever your child is diagnosed and is associated with better health in later life.

Insulin dose and timing

The exact times you monitor your child's blood glucose and give insulin each day will vary but will tend to follow a general pattern. For example, your child will need an insulin injection or dose around one or more of their mealtimes, and blood glucose checks either just before or 2 hours after meals.

The doses of insulin you need to give will vary over time. For up to about two years after diagnosis, your child may experience a period during which they will possibly need only small doses of insulin. Once this period is over, your child will need more insulin.

You may need to increase your child's insulin dose frequently when they have a growth spurt. You may also need to try different insulins and regimens from time to time to find one that best suits your child at their particular stage of development. Adjusting your child's insulin is an integral part of learning to live with diabetes, and your health professional will help you with this.

How to inject insulin

The procedure for injecting your child is the same as for an adult (see pp.56–57). Before giving an injection, ensure you wash your hands and have everything you need ready.

Try to stay calm and don't rush.

- Get your injection device ready, and fit a needle.
- Before injecting, you'll need to do an air-shot using 1 or 2 full or half units until insulin appears at the end of the needle.
- Make sure your child is sitting or being held firmly and comfortably and then inject into the nearest available site – the arm, abdomen, or bottom – using the pinch-up or direct technique you have been shown by your health professional.
- Keep the needle in the site for about 10 seconds and then withdraw it and place it safely away.
- After you've finished, comfort or distract your child.
- As soon as possible, safely dispose of the needle and return the injection device to where you normally keep it.

You may need to increase your child's insulin dose frequently when they have a growth spurt

Coping with resistance

There will be times when your child is unwilling to have an injection or to have their blood glucose checked. Think about how you encourage them to take care of other aspects of their health, such as toothbrushing, and try to incorporate diabetes care into their routine in the same way. Bear in mind that very young children may at first fiercely resist having an injection or blood glucose check but can be distracted easily immediately afterwards. Even if you sometimes feel guilty about giving your child an injection or doing a blood check when they are upset, consider the impact of any kind of reward you give afterwards. Having a cuddle, reading a book, or playing with a favourite toy together can help your child to link injection or blood monitoring time with a pleasurable experience, but rewards, such as new activities, new toys, or even food, can be difficult to deliver every day.

MONITORING OR INJECTING A RELUCTANT CHILD

- Explain what you are going to do and then do it immediately. Don't say that you'll do something "in 5 minutes" – this will increase any sense of anxiety.
- Hold your child firmly and securely on your knee as you carry out a blood glucose check or give an injection.
- Ask other family members to help if necessary.
- Allow your child to help if they want to (and are old enough).
- Cuddle and praise your child when the check or injection is finished.

▽ **Injecting insulin**
When injecting your child with insulin, it is important to change sites regularly to avoid potential problems with absorption.

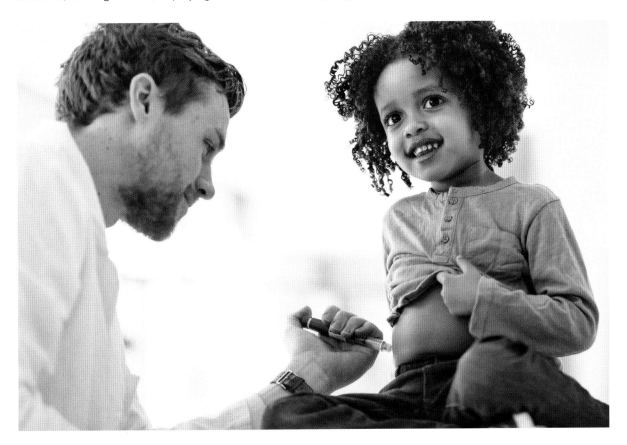

Babies and young children:
Dealing with hypoglycaemia

Hypoglycaemia is a side effect of insulin treatment so your child will have an episode from time to time, especially if you are achieving recommended blood glucose levels. However, if you are alert to signs of a hypo, you will be able to act quickly to help your child recover.

Recognizing warning signs

The signs of hypoglycaemia are individual for each child, but they tend to be the same each time so you will soon learn what they are. You also need to be aware that your child could have a severe hypo if they:

- Have been very physically active but haven't had less insulin or more food to compensate.
- Eat less than usual over several meals or feeds.
- Have had a recent increase in their dose of insulin.
- Become overheated.
- Are unwell, especially with vomiting.

A blood glucose check will confirm whether or not your child's blood glucose has fallen below 4 millimoles per litre (4 mmol/L), which means that they are hypoglycaemic. If you can't check and think your child is hypoglycaemic, it won't do any harm to give your baby a breastfeed or bottle feed, or your young child glucose or a sugary drink to raise their blood glucose. The sooner you treat a hypo, the sooner your child will recover.

A blood glucose check will tell you if **your child** is having an episode of **hypoglycaemia**

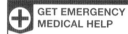

GET EMERGENCY MEDICAL HELP

- If treatment (see below and opposite) isn't working and your child continues to be hypoglycaemic.
- If your child becomes unconscious and there is nobody who has been shown how to inject glucagon or a glucagon kit is not available.
- If your child has difficulty breathing.
- If your child has a seizure. Do not restrain them but ensure they can't injure themselves.

Treating hypos

Because hypos can be unpredictable, it's useful to keep glucose tablets or gel, a sugary drink or a feed handy to treat them. You can also limit the risk of hypos by giving your child a feed, a carbohydrate snack at bedtime, or waking them for a feed or snack during the night. During the day, regular feeds or meals and snacks will help to balance insulin doses. If your child eats much less than usual at a mealtime or feed, you may need to reduce their next dose of insulin.

If you know that your child will be particularly active, you can give them more to eat or a reduced insulin dose beforehand. Extra activity can cause your child's blood glucose to fall several hours later, so you can give your child extra food after the activity to compensate.

TREATING A SEVERE HYPO

If severe hypoglycaemia is untreated, there is a risk that your child could become unconscious or have a seizure. If your child does have a seizure, it doesn't mean that they have epilepsy; it is the brain's reaction to a low glucose level. You will need to keep calm and take the following measures to help your child recover.

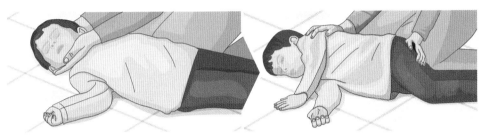

1 If your child is having a seizure, make sure their mouth is clear so that they can breathe. Ensure that they can't injure themselves and get emergency medical help.

2 If your child can breathe normally, lay them on their side or hold them with their head tilted back slightly to keep their airway clear. If your child is having a seizure, wait until it has stopped before doing this.

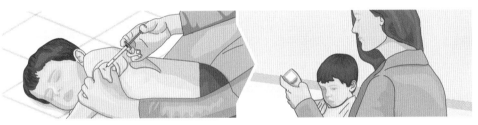

3 Prepare a glucagon injection (see p.67), or ask someone else to do so, and give it to your child in their arm, buttock, or leg. Don't try to give them anything to eat or drink.

4 When your child has regained consciousness, they might vomit as a result of the glucagon injection. Sit your child up and check their blood glucose as soon as it is practical to do so.

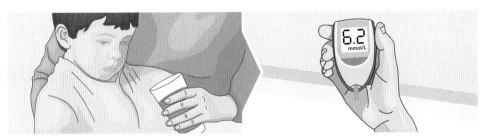

5 When your child is fully conscious and more alert, give them some food or drink containing carbohydrate or a feed to keep their blood glucose level raised.

6 Check your child's blood glucose level every 30 minutes until it is above 4 mmol/L and you are confident that they have recovered completely.

School-age children

Whether your child has recently been diagnosed with diabetes or has lived with it from a young age, their earlier school years – between the ages of about 5 and 12 – are a time of growing independence. They will understand more and can gradually learn to manage their diabetes themselves. However, support from you and your child's teachers is still essential so that your child can maintain good diabetes management and participate fully in all activities.

Diabetes, your child, and you

If your child already has diabetes when they reach school age, it is probably type 1 diabetes (see pp.12–13) and you will be giving them insulin. You will notice that their insulin requirement increases as they grow, and that you will also need to adjust the dosage more often in response to new activities at school or changes in the times at which they eat. If your child develops diabetes during their early school years, it is most likely to be type 1, although it may be type 2 (see pp.14–15) or MODY (maturity onset diabetes of the young, see pp.16–17), which, although still relatively rare, are becoming increasingly common in school-age children.

As a parent, it is important to balance caring for your child's diabetes and encouraging them to understand and manage it themselves without allowing the condition to dominate all your lives. Striking this balance can be challenging, but talking to your health professionals, helplines and online support groups, and particularly other parents of children with diabetes, can be useful not only for practical advice, but also for reassurance and psychological support.

Telling other people

In general, it is your decision who and how to tell other people about your child's diabetes. If their diagnosis is recent, you may want to inform others gradually as you become increasingly confident in dealing with the situation. Your relatives and close friends are likely to be the first people you tell, and they can be a valuable source of support for you and your child.

The main people who need to know about your child's diabetes are those who are directly involved in their care, such as your child's carer or school staff.

INVOLVING YOUR CHILD IN THEIR DIABETES

The following suggestions may help your child to understand their diabetes and become more actively engaged in managing it.

- Try to respond to any questions your child has about their diabetes as clearly and simply as you can.
- Be positive about any attempts your child makes to help with their diabetes, such as dialling the dose on an insulin pen.
- As your child gets older, encourage them to look at websites, apps, and books about diabetes, and allow them to choose suitable equipment that appeals to them.
- Your child's enthusiasm for managing their diabetes may come and go, so you should be prepared to take over if your child becomes reluctant to care for their diabetes themselves.

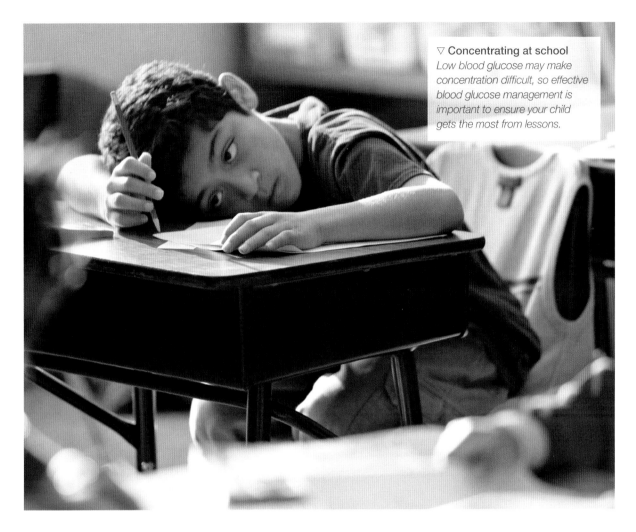

▽ **Concentrating at school**
Low blood glucose may make concentration difficult, so effective blood glucose management is important to ensure your child gets the most from lessons.

They will need to learn how your child's diabetes is managed, and also how to identify and respond to both low blood glucose levels (hypoglycaemia, see pp.164–165) and raised levels (hyperglycaemia, see pp.68–71), including giving emergency treatment and details of who to contact. The more information you can provide, the more confident other people will be in looking after your child. Your health professionals will be able to help you to advise and train caregivers and school staff about what to do for all activities and in all situations, such as school outings, and will also provide written guides and information.

A child with diabetes can do anything other children do, but blood glucose management is important to keep them healthy

School-age children:
Eating and drinking

Trying to keep to healthy eating guidelines for your child with diabetes will help them stay well. If your child has type 2 diabetes, which is rare compared with type 1, you will receive specialist individual advice on how to manage their food and, if necessary, their weight.

Healthy eating principles

The general principles of healthy eating (see pp.74–75) apply as much to your child with type 1 or type 2 diabetes as every other child. They should have several portions of fruit and vegetables every day, plus slow-acting carbohydrates, protein, and fat, plus sugar and salt but in small quantities only. Having regular drinks of water or sugar-free fluids is also important.

Children tend to need three healthy meals and three snacks a day, in order to balance their insulin, prevent hypos, and ensure they grow and develop properly. Your health professionals will offer information and support to help ensure that your child's food needs for their diabetes fit in with their overall health and wellbeing. They will also be able to help you be aware of the potential risk of eating difficulties (see p.179).

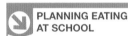

PLANNING EATING AT SCHOOL

You may need to ask the following questions to understand how best to plan your child's eating while at school:

- Are the children allowed to eat at break times?
- How often are breaks delayed?
- What time is lunch?
- When are sports lessons and how often are there extra or unplanned physical activities?
- What are the general eating arrangements on school trips?
- When is there extra food, such as for birthdays or celebrations?

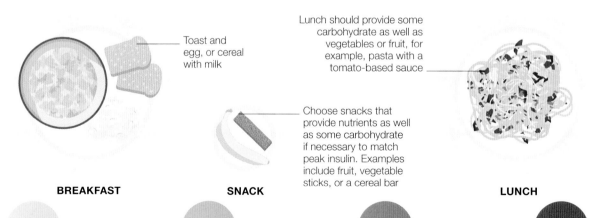

Toast and egg, or cereal with milk

Lunch should provide some carbohydrate as well as vegetables or fruit, for example, pasta with a tomato-based sauce

Choose snacks that provide nutrients as well as some carbohydrate if necessary to match peak insulin. Examples include fruit, vegetable sticks, or a cereal bar

BREAKFAST

SNACK

LUNCH

8.00   10.00   12.00   14.00

School and school trips
Your child can eat in the same way as other children, either meals that are provided at school or a packed lunch. You will need to discuss the timings of meals with the school, and any possible variations in those timings, so that you can arrange your child's insulin doses and ways to avoid them having a hypo.

On school trips, when meals might be earlier or later than usual, your child will need a few extra snacks and hypo supplies in case of delays. It's worth reminding your child not to eat all their snacks at once and not to share them with friends. Before your child goes on a school trip, check the following:
• The leaving and return times and whether these are likely to be delayed.
• Arrangements for snacks and meals.
• The name of the person in charge, and whether they are your child's usual teacher or someone else. If possible, ask for the person's mobile phone number.
• Arrangements for contacting parents if a problem occurs.

> **HEALTHY SNACK AND LUNCH IDEAS**
> • Filled wholegrain bagels, wraps, or finger rolls
> • Crumpets or breadsticks
> • Chopped mango, apple, or kiwi fruit
> • Wholegrain crisps or cereal bars
> • Low-sugar, low-fat yoghurt
> • Carrot, celery, and pepper sticks and hummus
> • Bowl of wholegrain cereal with milk

Eating out and parties
If eating out at a restaurant, a friend's house, or at a party is not a regular event, extra carbohydrate or high-fat food or more sugary treats on those occasions will not be harmful for your child. If their appetite or activity levels are unpredictable, you'll need to check their blood glucose afterwards to see if they need an extra snack, or alternatively, a small extra dose of insulin to bring their blood glucose down if it has risen. If celebrations are a regular part of your family's life, it may help to talk with your health professionals about specific plans to manage your child's diabetes on those occasions (see pp.88–89).

Meat or fish and vegetables; include carbohydrate, such as potatoes, rice, or flatbread

Hummus and vegetable sticks or a small sandwich

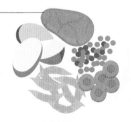
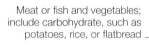

◁ **Meals and snacks**
Your child will need regular meals and snacks throughout the day. Choose nutritious foods from the main food groups. Some examples are shown here, but exact timings and food choices will vary with your child's preferences and routine.

A small snack before bedtime will help prevent a night-time hypo. Examples could be a glass of milk and a biscuit, or cereal with milk

SNACK 16.00   **DINNER** 18.00   **SNACK** 20.00   22.00

School-age children:
Blood glucose management

Making sure your child's blood glucose is managed effectively can be challenging as they grow up, spend time away from home at school, and become more independent. However, good blood glucose management is important too for their everyday wellbeing and to reduce the risk of long-term complications.

Recommended blood glucose levels

Good management of your child's diabetes means aiming for a blood glucose range of 4–7 millimoles per litre (mmol/L) most of the time and an HbA1c level (see p.31) of around 48 mmol/mol. Maintaining these levels means checking your child's blood glucose regularly and considering their treatment, activity, or food intake according to their levels. Making adjustments based on the pattern of blood glucose readings is more useful than acting on each individual one (see pp.150–151).

Responding to changes

As your child develops, their routine, activity levels, and rate of growth will change, which will affect their blood glucose levels and their insulin needs. In practice, this means that your child's blood glucose readings won't always be within the ideal range. A week or two outside this range from time to time won't do any harm, but consistently high blood glucose increases your child's risk of health problems when they get older.

A slightly raised blood glucose level won't necessarily make your child feel any different. They will only have symptoms, such as thirst or tiredness, with a blood glucose level of 10 mmol/L or higher. On the other hand, if they are tired or upset for other reasons, this can be confused with having a hypo. It can be hard to work out what to do without regular blood glucose checks, and so it can be helpful to use a method that is quick and easy, such as flash monitoring (see p.35 and p.37). This is also more comfortable for your child than the fingerprick method and can give you the information you need about the effect of any changes you have made to your child's insulin and/or food (see pp.48–51 for more information on adjusting insulin doses).

When your child starts school, their diabetes management will need to be adjusted

MANAGING YOUR CHILD'S INSULIN TREATMENT

- If you can't predict how much or when your child will eat, an insulin pump or a different insulin regimen may be helpful.

- Keep in mind that it's the overall management of your child's diabetes that matters, not a single blood glucose reading.

- Make sure that your child hasn't had so many snacks or drinks that they can't eat at mealtimes. If you're worried about your child having a hypo between meals or at school, you may need to adjust their insulin or medication doses instead.

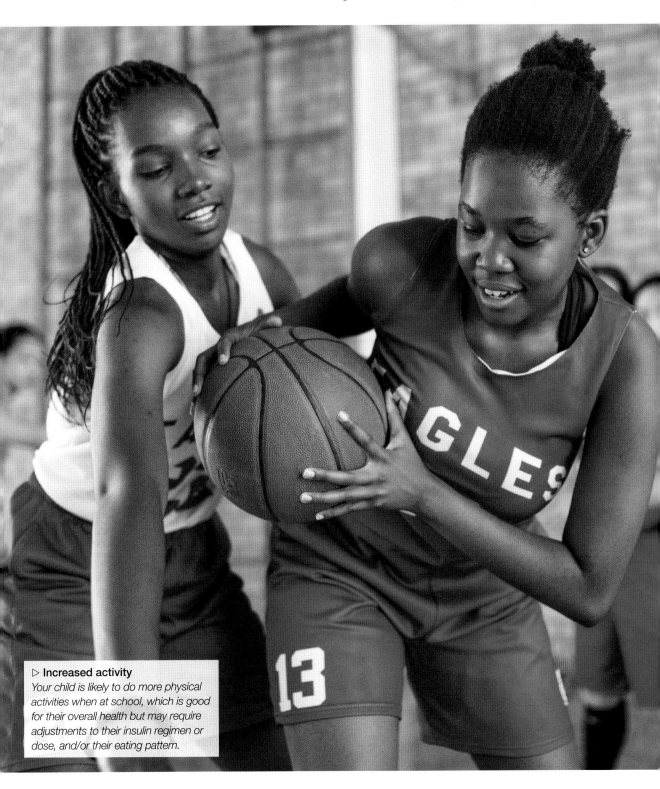

▷ **Increased activity**
Your child is likely to do more physical activities when at school, which is good for their overall health but may require adjustments to their insulin regimen or dose, and/or their eating pattern.

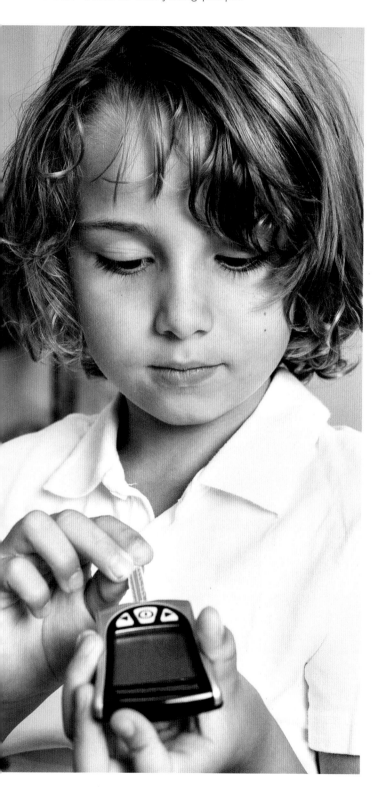

School-age children:
Blood glucose and insulin

Managing you child's blood glucose checks and insulin can be difficult, but there are ways of fitting them into the daily routine. Your health professional will be able to advise you about this and will also be able to help school staff with managing your child's diabetes.

Fitting diabetes into daily life

Insulin and blood glucose checks are an essential part of your child's life. Treating them like any other daily activity can help your child learn the importance of caring for their diabetes and preventing problems from occurring (see panel, opposite).

The practical processes of doing blood glucose checks and injecting insulin are the same as for an adult (see pp.36–37 for checking blood glucose, and pp.56–57 for injecting insulin). In time, the practicalities of diabetes care will become an integral part of your child's daily routine. However, like other routine daily activities, such as brushing your teeth or handwashing,

◁ **Helping your child become involved**
Supporting your child in choosing a new item of diabetes equipment, such as a blood glucose meter, flash monitor, or injection device, can encourage them to become involved in their diabetes.

sometimes an aspect of diabetes care may be overlooked or done later than usual. It is important to accept that this will happen from time to time and to realize that it is the overall management of your child's diabetes that is most important, rather than any single event. Keeping this in mind and passing it on to your child can help them to develop a healthy perspective on their diabetes as they grow older.

Important considerations in managing your child's diabetes are to try to avoid hypos and to take prompt action when they do occur (see pp.164–165). The possibility of your child having a hypo can be worrying, especially when they are away from you, doing something new, or at night. Talking over your concerns with your health professional will help to reassure you and ensure you have all the information you need to avoid and deal with hypos.

Involving your child

You will know the best time to start involving your child in their own diabetes care. In general, involving them as much as possible in, for example, working out what their blood glucose levels mean and what changes you need to make to their insulin (or other medication if they have type 2 diabetes or MODY), activity, or food, will help them towards taking responsibility in the longer term. There will be times when your child is not interested, reluctant, or wants to change the timings of checks or injections. Thinking in advance about these situations and discussing them with your health professionals and other parents will help you to find ways of dealing with them when they do occur.

As your **child** gets older, you can start to **involve them** in their **diabetes care**

Involving your child's school

Your child may need to have blood glucose checks and insulin at school, so you will need to discuss with school staff and your health professional how these can be managed successfully. For example, it may be necessary to train school staff how to carry out these procedures. When your child is old enough and feels confident, they will be able to manage their monitoring and insulin themselves, although they may still need support from school staff.

In turn, teachers and other staff will be able to give you information about how your child is coping at school, so together you can find ways to encourage them or address any difficulties your child is experiencing.

PREVENTING PROBLEMS

- Injecting insulin constantly in the same site causes lumps, called lipohypertrophy (or lipos), and also means that insulin is not absorbed properly. Change the site of their injection or cannula regularly and teach your child to do this themselves.

- Flash monitoring (see p.35 and p.37) can help to make blood glucose checks easier and painless. If you are not already using a flash monitor, talk with your health professional about trying one out.

- If your child has or develops fears about injections, blood glucose monitoring, hypos, or anything diabetes-related, take these seriously and explore them, with the help of your health professionals, if necessary.

School-age children:
Dealing with hypoglycaemia

When your child starts school, they will be in a new environment and have a new routine. You will naturally be concerned about the possibility of them having a hypo when you are not there, but you can help to reduce this worry by making sure that your child and the school or activity staff know how to recognize the signs of a hypo and, if your child does have one, how to treat it quickly and effectively,

Recognizing hypoglycaemia in a school-age child

The indications that your child is having a hypo – a blood glucose level below 4 millimoles per litre (mmol/L) – are individual to each child, but will be familiar to you as the child's parent. Encouraging your child to recognize the signs of a hypo themselves and to ask for help before it becomes worse is a good start. Sometimes, however, your child will be unaware of the signs or can't say how they feel, so their teachers or activity staff also need to be aware of your child's individual signs. Ideally, a blood glucose check will be carried out to confirm hypoglycaemia, but if it isn't possible to do a check, it won't do any harm to treat what seems to be a hypo straight away. Your health professional can help with teaching the school and other staff about hypos and how to deal with them.

Treating a hypo in a school-age child

The treatment for hypoglycaemia in a school-age child is the same as that for an adult (see pp.66–67). In the early stages, a hypo can usually be treated effectively by giving your child something to eat or drink that is high in sugar. When your child is old enough, teach them to carry something sugary at all times and eat it as soon as they recognize their hypo signs.

If a hypo becomes more severe, your child cannot swallow, or they become unconscious, they will need to be given a glucagon injection to raise their blood glucose. The injection will need to be given by you (if you are available at short notice), a member of the school or activity staff who has been shown how to inject, or, if nobody who is familiar with the procedure is available, by emergency medical personnel.

POSSIBLE SIGNS OF A HYPO IN A SCHOOL-AGE CHILD

Although the specific pattern of signs varies from child to child, they tend to be similar each time for a particular child. A detailed list of possible signs and symptoms is given on pp.64–65; however, common indications of a hypo in a school-age child may include:

- Unusual naughtiness, argumentativeness, restlessness, or silence
- Difficulty concentrating
- Sleepiness
- Loss of coordination
- Sweating
- Paler than normal skin

Avoiding hypos

Although you will want to protect your child against hypos, try to avoid the temptation to keep their blood glucose consistently raised (above 10 mmol/L) in an effort to prevent them. This tends not to be a reliable way of avoiding hypos, because insulin levels in your child's blood and the amount of energy they use may vary a lot during the day. In addition, a high blood glucose level can produce unpleasant symptoms as well as put your child at risk of health complications in the future.

Hypos can also occur some time after your child has been physically active as the muscles replace the energy they have used by taking glucose from the bloodstream, and because your child's insulin will still be working. It's important that your child is active because of the health benefits of exercise, so to reduce the risk of hypos, try changing the time of your child's insulin injection or reducing their dose before any planned activity. If their activity is unplanned, give your child an extra carbohydrate snack afterwards. If the activity lasts longer than about an hour, your child may need extra glucose in the form of a sugary drink or sweets during the activity, too.

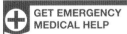

GET EMERGENCY MEDICAL HELP

- If the treatment for a hypo (see pp.66–67) isn't working and your child continues to be hypoglycaemic.

- If your child becomes unconscious and there is nobody to inject glucagon or a glucagon kit is not available.

- If your child has difficulty breathing.

- If your child has a seizure.

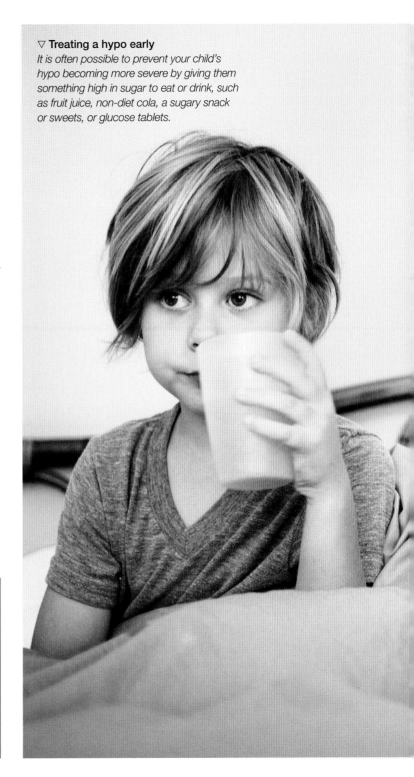

▽ **Treating a hypo early**
It is often possible to prevent your child's hypo becoming more severe by giving them something high in sugar to eat or drink, such as fruit juice, non-diet cola, a sugary snack or sweets, or glucose tablets.

Teenagers and young adults

Adolescence is a time of change and challenge: a teenager with diabetes not only has friendships, exams, the effects of hormones, and growing independence to deal with, but also blood glucose management. As a parent, you want to be supportive. As a teenager, you need to cope with your feelings and take care of your diabetes in ways that suit your lifestyle.

Diabetes, your teenager, and you

Having diabetes can complicate your teenager's life and cause you worry as a parent, but there are ways of working together to reduce any stress. As a parent, you may be tempted to try to be in control of your teenager's diabetes, but seeing it as their condition and increasing their responsibility for it can be a more supportive and successful strategy. Teenagers still need, and tend to respond to, rules and boundaries, even though they might argue about them. Being firm and consistent, and treating diabetes care as you would any other aspect of your teenager's life, can help. For example, you might agree that your teenager performs a certain number of blood checks per day or that they attend clinic visits regularly. The more you involve your teenager in making decisions that affect them, the more likely it is that they will achieve what has been agreed.

How teenagers treat their diabetes varies, but it is likely to be similar to the way in which they treat other aspects of their lives. A teenager who is doing anything that is important in managing their diabetes is likely to respond well to praise and encouragement. However, they may also see their diabetes as setting them apart from their friends and so try to make it less obvious by ignoring it or doing little in the way of monitoring or eating healthily. If you are worried that your teenager is not doing enough to manage their diabetes and none of your suggestions seems to work, they may be more receptive to friends or other family members, so ask for support from anyone you think will help. You can also contact your diabetes health professional for teenagers and young adults.

INTERACTING WITH YOUR TEENAGER

- Help your teenager plan how to look after their diabetes in every kind of situation.

- Encourage your teenager to come up with their own solutions to problems with diabetes management – they will learn more by experimenting than by simply following instructions.

- Remind your teenager often that you respect, love, and support them.

- Try to allow your teenager to join in with what their friends are doing.

- Try to say "yes" rather than refuse on account of your teenager's diabetes.

- When you ask questions about your teenager's diabetes, try to make it part of an ongoing conversation rather than the sole focus.

- Listen calmly to anything they say.

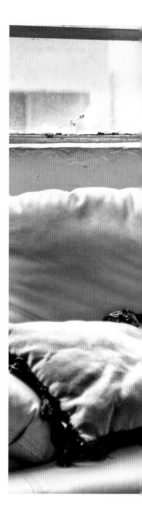

△ **Talking to your teenager**
Good communication involves listening as well as talking, so it is important to give your teenager time to talk. Even if you have disagreements or arguments, it helps to remain calm and to keep lines of communication open.

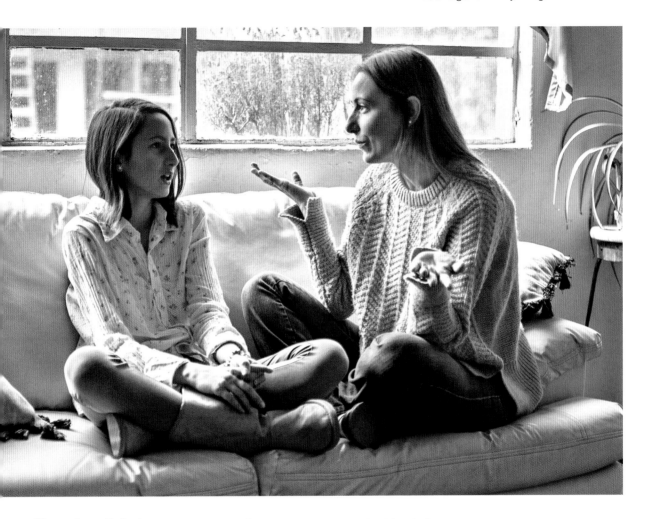

Changing diabetes management

Diabetes management for teenagers with type 1 or type 2 diabetes, or MODY (see pp.16–17) is personalized for each individual and will need to change as they grow and develop, and as their circumstances change. For example, it is likely that the effect of hormones will increase the amount of insulin a teenager with type 1 diabetes needs as they go through adolescence. In addition, the pressures of exams or starting work, developing sexually, and possibly experimenting with alcohol or drugs will also affect their blood glucose.

As a result, regular blood glucose monitoring and contact with your teenager's diabetes health professional are crucial to ensure that their diabetes is managed effectively. The health professional can also advise about new technology that may it easier for your teenager to manage their diabetes.

Good **management** of your **teenager's diabetes** is important to keep them **healthy** and help **avoid complications** in the future

Teenagers and young adults:
Dealing with your feelings

When you have diabetes as young person, you may experience a range of feelings, both positive and negative. If you have constant negative feelings, your healthcare professional can help. Some of the best people to understand your situation are others with diabetes, and meeting them in person or online can be reassuring.

Your feelings about diabetes

However long you have had diabetes and whatever type you have, you will have a range of feelings at different times, from positive, such as acceptance or feeling motivated, to negative, for example, anger, resentment, guilt, or even embarrassment. It's important to know that these are to be expected, because diabetes is a difficult and demanding condition that can sometimes seriously disrupt your life.

If stress related to your diabetes becomes an issue from time to time, try using coping strategies (see opposite). However, if you constantly have negative feelings that make you avoid caring for your diabetes, you should share this with someone else, such as your parents or a close relative, a friend's parent, a diabetes health professional or helpline, or a school or college counsellor, so that they can help you.

Your friends and your feelings

You may be concerned that your friends will think differently about you if you tell them you have diabetes. You may even have experience of people being unkind simply because of your diabetes, which may put you off telling others or ignoring your diabetes. If you do want to tell a friend, thinking about what to say in advance can help to make it easier. Your real friends will be genuinely interested, accepting, and supportive. If you are being bullied or hassled by anyone at school, college, or work because of your diabetes, it is important to report this to a teacher, tutor, or employer.

Peer support

Support from other young people with diabetes is one of the best ways to help you feel you are not alone or different and that you can cope with your diabetes. Meeting others in a similar situation means that you can share the experiences, ups and downs of life with diabetes, and practical ways of dealing with challenges. Your local area may have face-to-face activities or diabetes

---

⊕ GET EMERGENCY MEDICAL HELP

- If you are persistently depressed, tearful, or anxious and/or withdraw from or avoid social interactions.
- If you are becoming anxious about food and eating and are avoiding your diabetes management.
- If you are having thoughts of harming yourself or somebody else.

education classes that bring you together, and there are also many online and social media forums, discussions, and events to participate in. As well as providing practical help and support, these events are also an opportunity to meet new people and make new friends.

Mental health

Diabetes may sometimes cause specific psychological issues, such as diabetes-related distress and burnout (see p.111) or diabetes-specific fear of hypoglycaemia (see p.176). Your diabetes health professionals will be able to identify these problems and offer help. However, you may already have a mental health condition when you are diagnosed with diabetes, or you may develop one after diagnosis. Your treatment for these additional conditions will continue or be the same as for anyone else, and, if necessary, your diabetes management will be adjusted. It can be difficult to manage more than one condition, and you will be offered extra emotional support and practical help.

Support from other young people with diabetes can help you feel that you can cope with your diabetes

Talk with or message other people with diabetes. Sometimes, simply sharing your feelings with others in the same situation can help to reduce your stress.

Try to take regular exercise. This will not only benefit your physical health but can also help to improve feelings of low mood.

Listen to music or podcasts, watch videos, or visit websites you find uplifting and enjoyable.

Remind yourself that having diabetes is not your fault and that you are doing your best. You may find it helpful to list your positive achievements in caring for your diabetes.

Think about refreshing the way you manage your diabetes, perhaps by using an insulin pump, a different insulin regimen, or a new form of blood glucose monitoring.

Talk with your health professional. This is especially important if other measures haven't worked or if you are experiencing persistent negative thoughts or feelings.

△ **Dealing with diabetes stress**
Occasional periods of diabetes stress are normal and you can often deal with them effectively by using one or more of the coping strategies outlined above.

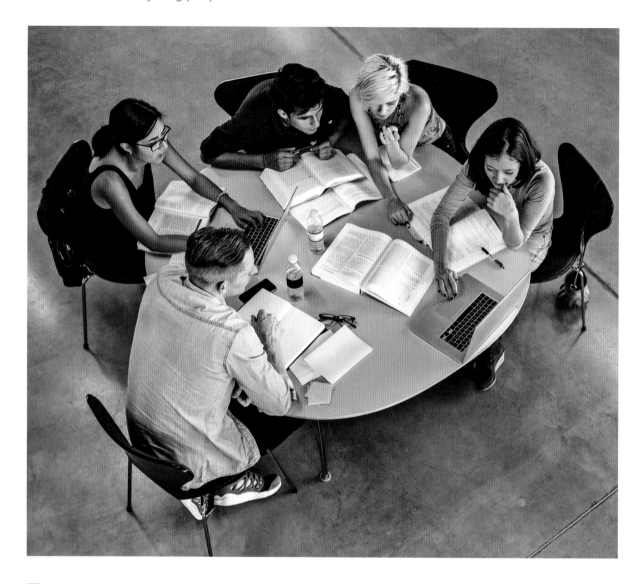

Teenagers and young adults:
Getting on with your life

There are few things you cannot do with diabetes. Modern, flexible treatment regimens and new technology have made it easier to manage your diabetes so that can fit in with your life. As a young adult, you will take more responsibility for managing your diabetes yourself, but your health professionals will help so you can do this successfully and with the least inconvenience.

△ **Long study periods**
When you are studying, it can be easy to forget to take your medication or eat. Setting up a reminder on your smartphone or watch can be useful to ensure that you don't miss food or medication times.

Your diabetes care*

If you were a child when first diagnosed, as a teenager you will be offered a transition service (known as young adult care) between the child and adult diabetes care services. If you were already a young adult when diagnosed, you will probably enter the adult service directly. However, there is no specific age at which you transition, it will depend on factors such as where you live and if you and your existing healthcare professionals think you are ready. Transitioning means learning to manage your diabetes independently, and the healthcare professionals will ensure you have the knowledge, skills, and equipment to do so successfully.

When you move to adult care, certain aspects of your diabetes care will change:

• Your healthcare professionals will be different.

• Your contact for emergency help between appointments will change.

• The time, location, and number of your diabetes healthcare appointments will change. You will be offered regular discussions and health checks as well as an annual review (see pp.142–143).

• Your recommended targets, such as your blood glucose levels and HbA1c (see p.31), might be adjusted.

You can continue to bring your parents or friends to appointments if you feel you need their support. However, your new healthcare professionals will talk to you directly about your diabetes.

If you have type 1 diabetes, you will need to take insulin (see pp.42–51). If you have type 2 diabetes or prediabetes, you may be taking tablets (see pp.58–59) or insulin or a combination of both. For all types, you will need to check your blood glucose regularly (see pp.36–39).

The practicalities of looking after your diabetes may make you feel self-conscious or different from your friends but choosing the equipment or medication regimen that is right for you can often help. Your health professional will be able to offer advice so you can find the right solution for you personally.

Managing illness

An important aspect of starting to manage your diabetes yourself is learning how to deal with illness (see pp.124–125). This is because illness can make your blood glucose rise very high and put you at risk of potentially serious complications (see hyperglycaemia, pp.68–71). Continuing to take your medication and getting medical advice sooner rather than later when you are ill will help to prevent your diabetes making you even more unwell.

School, study, and work

How you manage your diabetes at school, university, or at work will depend on your timetable or routine. As these change, you may need to change the type or timings of your medication, blood glucose monitoring, or eating patterns. Stressful times, such as exams or job interviews, are likely to make your blood glucose rise, and prolonged periods of studying or work may mean that you miss meals. Having your diabetes equipment and hypo remedies with you at all times is a good way to make sure you are well prepared.

As a **young adult**, you will learn how to **manage** your **diabetes independently**

If an organization has rules about eating, drinking, or medication that make your diabetes management difficult, your health professionals will be able to help you to resolve the issue. For example, they may be able to suggest adjusting your diabetes regimen to better fit your routine. They can also inform you of your legal situation regarding discrimination and diabetes.

Moving away from home

Leaving home involves a change of routine and responsibility, so it can be exciting but it may also cause you concern. If you are going to live independently, it is important to remember the following points:

● You will need to register with a local GP, who can refer you to the specialist diabetes service for a new area. This will enable you to continue to get your prescriptions and ensure you have advice and help when you need them.

● If you are going away to study, you should tell the establishment that you have diabetes. They may be able to help with any special arrangements you need.

● You will be completely responsible for your food. Make sure you have enough carbohydrate foods and hypo treatments for when you need them.

● If you share accommodation, keep hypo treatments in your room as well as the kitchen.

● Tell a flatmate or friend you see frequently about your diabetes and how to treat a hypo (see pp.66–67) in case you're unable to treat yourself.

Going out, holidays, and travel

Some entertainment venues have restrictions on the type and size of items allowed, although these are often relaxed for medical equipment. Finding out your venue's policy and planning in advance of your visit – for example, by obtaining written confirmation of your diabetes

▽ **Attending events**
Your diabetes needn't mean you have to avoid events such as music concerts or festivals. However, you should make sure you take all the medication, food, and equipment you will need while there.

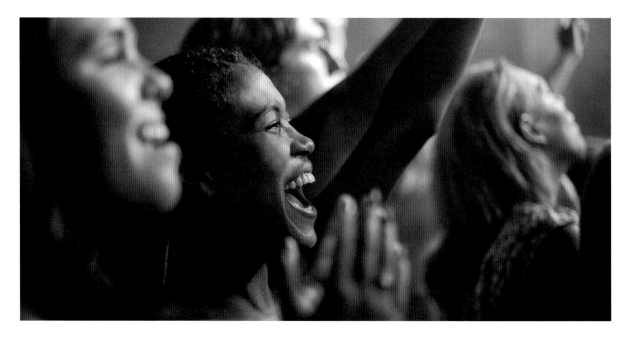

from your health professional – will ensure that nothing prevents you from enjoying yourself. It is also advisable to take your ID as proof of your age.

Having holidays with friends and even spending long periods travelling are all possible with the proper planning (see pp.116–117). Similarly, having diabetes will not prevent you from learning to drive and getting a licence when you are old enough, although, depending on your diabetes and its management, you may have to inform the relevant authorities beforehand (see pp.114–115).

Drinking alcohol

Having diabetes doesn't mean you can't drink alcohol – when you're old enough to do so legally. However, alcohol can have extra effects because of your diabetes treatment, especially if you use insulin or insulin-stimulating medication (see pp.58–59). The main effects are that hypo symptoms may be similar to those of being drunk, so you may not be able to recognize and treat a hypo effectively. In addition, your body cannot recover well from a hypo when you have had a lot of alcohol, so a hypo may be prolonged and severe, which can lead to you losing consciousness. (For more information about alcohol, see pp.86–87.)

Relationships and sex

When and how you tell your partner that you have diabetes is your decision. If you are sexually active, it is important to make your partner aware of your diabetes because sex is a form of physical activity and can affect your blood glucose level, potentially causing a hypo. In a heterosexual relationship, using contraception when a female partner has diabetes is particularly important, unless you are planning a pregnancy, because their blood glucose at the time of conception has a large effect on the health of a baby (see pp.118–119).

SMOKING AND RECREATIONAL DRUGS

Smoking has a wide range of adverse health effects but it is particularly harmful for people with diabetes. Recreational drugs are also a particular health risk when you have diabetes.

Smoking

Having diabetes puts you at increased risk of heart and circulation problems, and smoking increases this risk significantly. The nicotine in tobacco smoke is also highly addictive. Smoking e-cigarettes (vaping) is commonly thought to be less harmful, but the fumes still contain nicotine and the safety of vaping has not been established. The best way to minimize the risk is not to start smoking or vaping. If you already do so, you can get support from health professionals to stop.

Drugs

Recreational drugs may be harmful in themselves. For people with diabetes, there is the additional risk that a drug may mask the effects of a hypo and/or affect your alertness, which can make you forget to eat or take your diabetes medication. The safest course of action is simply to avoid taking any such substances.

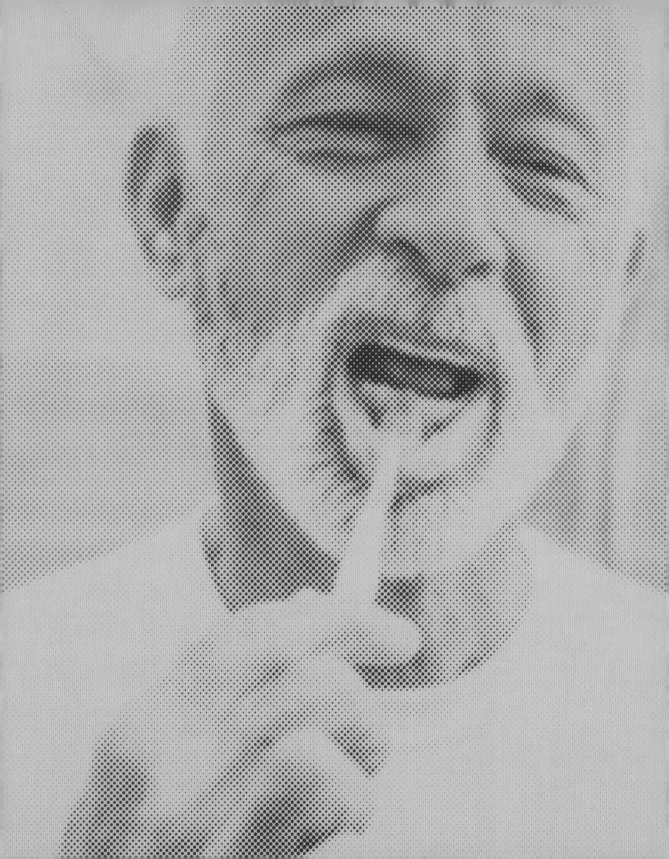

Dealing with complications

Psychological problems

It is normal for diabetes to have an impact on you emotionally (see pp.110–111), but for some people the condition may lead to psychological problems, such as anxiety, depression, or specific fears. These may affect many areas of your everyday life, including how you manage your diabetes, which is why it is important to obtain professional help.

Fear of hypoglycaemia

Many people with diabetes have episodes of hypoglycaemia (low blood glucose, see pp.62–67) from time to time and deal with them without major issues. However, some people develop a severe fear of hypos and take unwise measures to avoid them. For example, they may reduce or even stop their diabetes medication so that their blood glucose remains high, which increases the risk of future physical complications. They may also check their blood glucose far more frequently than necessary. If you have an extreme fear of hypos, your health professional can help by discussing the problem and, together,

you can make a plan to reduce your fear. This might include a refresher course to help your confidence in dealing with hypos, or using a continuous glucose monitor so that you can see your blood glucose level clearly at all times.

Your health professional may also refer you for specialist psychological help, such as cognitive behavioural therapy (CBT, see panel, opposite). You may need a combination of treatments to successfully reduce your fear of hypos.

Fear of physical complications

Being extremely worried about developing serious complications of diabetes can sometimes become overwhelming. Your fear might lead you to keep your blood glucose very low, putting you at risk of hypos or losing warning signs of them. You may become anxious about any rise in your blood glucose, even if it remains within your target range, or you may even feel it's not worth looking after your diabetes at all.

▷ **Discussing your issues**
It is important to be discuss any psychological issues you have with your healthcare professional sooner rather than later so that together you can find a way to resolve them before they lead to potentially more serious problems.

SOURCES OF HELP

If you have a psychological problem, there are many sources of help and support available, including:

- Your diabetes specialist health professional, who can provide information, practical help and encouragement, treatment, and refer you to specialist services.

- Diabetes organizations, online forums, and social media, which can give useful information about how other people with diabetes cope in situations similar to yours.

- Mental health organizations, which can provide with information and peer support related to your particular problem.

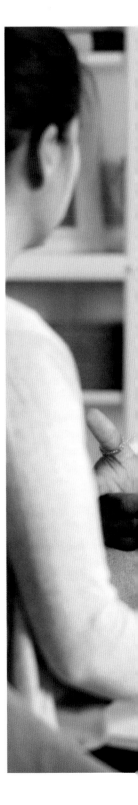

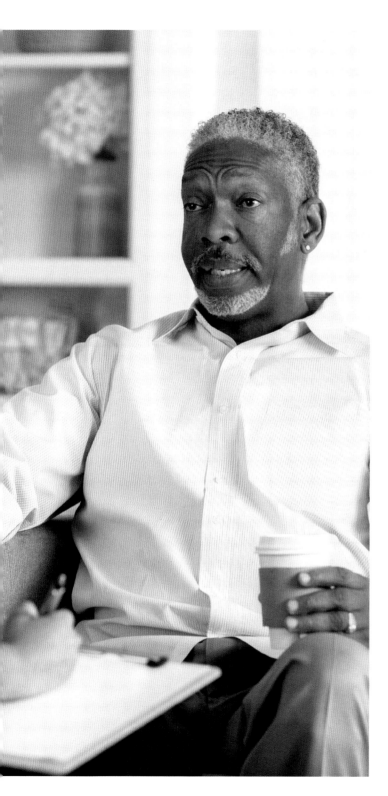

COGNITIVE BEHAVIOURAL THERAPY

Commonly known as CBT, cognitive behavioural therapy helps you recognize and understand your distressing thought patterns and behaviour and shows ways to consciously adopt more helpful thinking styles and behaviour. When you take part in CBT, you will probably be asked to record your thoughts, feelings, and behaviour. During a therapy session, these are analysed to help identify inappropriate ones. The therapist will then help you to develop techniques for changing them.

Talking with your health professional is the first step to helping you with your fear. They will be able to give you information about how complications develop, give insight into your personal risk of complications, and give practical advice on how to reduce your risk. They can also help you to find ways of minimizing your fear and its impact on your life, such as getting support from family and friends, and, if necessary, can arrange for you to have specialist psychological therapy.

Concern about injections, fingerpricks, or using insulin

You may be concerned about first starting to use insulin, injections, or fingerprick blood glucose checks, particularly if you have only recently been diagnosed with diabetes. This may lead you to avoid medical appointments and continue to live with raised blood glucose levels. If this is the case, you are at risk of becoming unwell with an infection, or with diabetic ketoacidosis

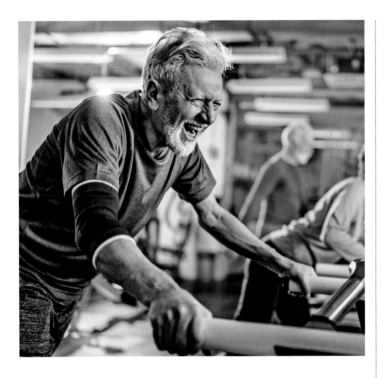

△ **Boosting your mood**
Regular exercise can help to relieve anxiety and boost your mood if you are depressed. Choose a type of exercise you enjoy so that you stay motivated to do it regularly.

(DKA), or hyperosmolar hyperglycaemic state (HHS). DKA and HHS (see p.71) are potentially life-threatening and need urgent medical treatment.

If you have any concerns, share them with your diabetes healthcare professional. Not only will they be able to answer your questions and provide reassurance, they will also give you the opportunity of experiencing a demonstration injection or fingerprick blood glucose check, so that you know the reality. They may also suggest that you use the new equipment or treatment for a trial period, with an evaluation at the end, to help you gain confidence and alleviate your concerns.

An extreme fear of needles – needle phobia – is rare. If you have it, you may experience severe anxiety symptoms at the sight of needles or blood, such as palpitations, sweating, nausea, and

fainting. Having this phobia will make your diabetes difficult to manage and you will need specialist psychological help, which your diabetes health professional will be able to arrange.

Anxiety

Occasional bouts of anxiety are common, but if you experience them regularly for six months or more, you can benefit from professional treatment because anxiety can affect all aspects of life, including diabetes. Typical symptoms of anxiety include feeling nervous, being unable to relax, finding it difficult to concentrate, repetitive worrying thoughts, and sleep problems. You may also have panic attacks: sudden episodes of intense fear in a particular situation, such as being in an enclosed space.

Your health professional will be able to help, by discussing and assessing your symptoms, prescribing anti-anxiety medication, and/or referring you for specialist therapy, such as cognitive behavioural therapy (see p.177). They will also be able to advise on how to deal with anxiety on a day-to-day basis, for example, with exercise, relaxation, or breathing activities, and may be able to suggest ways in which you can adjust your diabetes treatment regimen temporarily to make it less stressful.

Depression

This is a common problem for people with diabetes, probably at least partly due to the continual need to manage the condition. Being depressed can stop you looking after yourself and managing your diabetes properly, which is why it is important to recognize the symptoms and obtain professional help.

Typical symptoms of depression include feeling low, taking less interest or pleasure in activities you usually find enjoyable, tiredness, irritability, difficulty concentrating, problems sleeping, and feeling worthless, guilty, or hopeless. Some of these are similar to those of high blood glucose (see pp.68–71) or low blood glucose (see pp.62–67). However, with depression, the symptoms persist long-term, whereas with the other conditions symptoms improve once the underlying blood-glucose problem has been corrected.

If you suspect you have depression, you can consult your healthcare professional for assessment, and for treatment and/or referral to a specialist, such as a psychotherapist. Treatment may involve a talking therapy, such as cognitive behavioural therapy (CBT, see p.177), medication, or both. Your health professional will also be able to help you with managing your diabetes while you are depressed.

Eating problems

When you have diabetes, you need to pay extra attention to food but if you regularly have concerns about food and eating, such as restricting your food to manage your weight, this is known as disordered eating. Certain specific eating behaviours are also considered to be eating disorders (see panel, above right). You may regularly use less insulin than you need in order to lose weight. Known as insulin restriction, this may lead to diabetic ketoacidosis or hyperosmolar hyperglycaemic state (see p.71).

Eating problems make diabetes harder to manage and may make physical complications more likely

---

FEATURES OF EATING DISORDERS

The main eating disorders are anorexia nervosa (commonly known just as anorexia), bulimia nervosa (or just bulimia), and binge-eating disorder. They are all characterized by particular attitudes to food, but have different behavioural features.

DISORDER	COMMON FEATURES
Anorexia	Preoccupation with body weight and size; severe restriction of calorie intake; extreme weight loss; excessive exercising; use of laxatives and/or appetite suppressants.
Bulimia	Binge eating followed by self-induced vomiting and/or laxative use; episodes tend to occur regularly, such as weekly; guilt after binge eating; physical weakness.
Binge-eating disorder	Eating very large amounts in a short time; eating secretly and/or trying to hide how much food is eaten; feeling a loss of control when eating large amounts; often, weight gain.

Psychological issues could potentially affect your ability to manage your diabetes

to develop. Your health professional will ask about your eating during your health reviews. They will also share any concerns they have about your weight or eating and, if necessary, will offer you specialist help, for example, from a dietitian and/or therapist. They will continue to help you manage your diabetes during any specialist treatment.

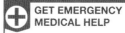 **GET EMERGENCY MEDICAL HELP**

- If you have thoughts of self-harm or suicide.
- If you have symptoms of diabetic ketoacidosis or hyperosmolar hyperglycaemic state (see p.71).

Eye conditions

Longstanding diabetes or raised blood glucose can cause damage to your eyes' blood supply. This condition is called retinopathy and, if untreated and progressive, may lead to loss of vision. Regular eye checks are vital to enable early detection and treatment, and careful diabetes management can prevent the condition from worsening and affecting vision. Cataracts are also more common if you have diabetes but can be treated to prevent visual impairment.

Retinopathy

The retina is the light-sensitive layer of the eye. To function properly, it needs a plentiful supply of blood, provided by a network of tiny vessels. In long-term diabetes, constant raised blood glucose and/or high blood pressure may lead to retinopathy, in which these vessels become weak and fragile.

Stages of retinopathy

There are three main stages of retinopathy:
● **Background retinopathy** In this early stage, blood vessels bulge and leak blood. These bulges, known as microaneurysms, appear as small red dots during

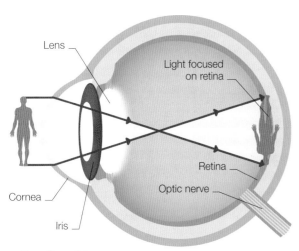

△ **Function of the eye**
Light entering the eye is focused by the cornea and lens onto the retina. Cells here convert the light to nerve impulses; these pass along the optic nerve to the brain, where they are interpreted as an image.

examination of the retina. Yellowish spots called exudates (formed of substances leaked from the blood vessels), and white areas known as cotton-wool spots (where blood vessels have closed down) may also develop. Many people who have had type 1 diabetes for about 20 years have some background retinopathy but it does not always progress further.
● **Preproliferative retinopathy** In this stage (also sometimes known as non-proliferative retinopathy), the damage is progressing. Eye examinations reveal many microaneurysms, exudates, and cotton-wool spots. New, fragile blood vessels start to form on the retina to replace the ones that have closed down.
● **Proliferative retinopathy** If preproliferative retinopathy is not treated, many more fragile new blood vessels form on the retina. These vessels may bleed into the eye, causing reduced vision.

Causes

Retinopathy can result from longstanding diabetes or a blood glucose level that has been consistently raised for years. High blood pressure can also be a contributing factor. Pregnancy may cause retinopathy to appear or to progress more rapidly than it would otherwise.

Symptoms and diagnosis

Retinopathy does not usually cause symptoms until the proliferative stage, when it starts to impair vision. It may affect one or both of your eyes and there may be partial or total loss of vision.

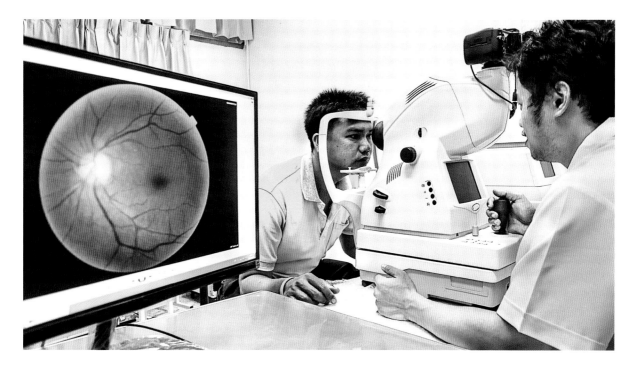

You will be offered retinal screening to check for retinopathy at least once a year. This involves taking photographs of your retina to check for signs of damage. If you already have retinal damage or you are pregnant, you will be offered eye tests more often. These may include tests of visual acuity, in which you are asked to read letters of diminishing size; photographs of your retina; and a direct visual examination of your retina using an instrument called an ophthalmoscope. If you already have advanced retinopathy, you may also have specialized imaging to pinpoint the affected area of your retina.

Complications

If retinopathy is treated early, its progress can often be halted. However, without treatment, retinopathy can progress and lead to complications such as maculopathy, vitreous haemorrhage, retinal detachment, or glaucoma (see p.183).

Maculopathy affects the macula, the small central area of the retina that is responsible for high-resolution colour vision. It is more common if you have type 2 diabetes. In maculopathy, the tiny

△ **Retinal photography**

Digital photographs of your retina may be taken to check for retinopathy. In the images, the blood vessels can be seen as a network branching from the optic disc, where the optic nerve starts.

blood vessels around the macula may leak, leading to a build-up of fluid; the blood supply to the macula may be reduced; or fatty deposits may accumulate on the macula. In all of these, the macula becomes damaged, which may threaten your eyesight.

Vitreous haemorrhage is bleeding into the vitreous humour, the jelly-like substance that fills the back of the eye. It occurs if you have proliferative retinopathy and the new blood vessels in your retina bleed profusely. You may suddenly lose a large part of your vision, although this is usually temporary as the blood is gradually reabsorbed.

Retinal detachment, in which your retina becomes separated from the underlying layers of the eye, may occur a few weeks after a vitreous haemorrhage. Without treatment, it can cause permanent damage to your vision.

Prevention and treatment

The best way to prevent retinopathy from developing or progressing is careful long-term blood glucose management and effective treatment of high blood pressure (see pp.192–193), if you also have this condition. It is also important to attend your appointments for eye examinations, including retinal screening.

Treatment of retinopathy depends on how advanced the condition is. If you have background retinopathy, you don't need any treatment, but your eyes need to be examined every 6 months. If you have a high blood glucose level that suddenly reduces because you are intensifying your treatment, your retinopathy may actually worsen; lowering your blood glucose level over a few months rather than weeks can prevent this.

If you have preproliferative or proliferative retinopathy, you will probably be offered laser treatment to target the fragile new blood vessels in the damaged area of your retina. Maculopathy may be treated with lasers, or sometimes with injections of medication into the eye. You may also be offered laser treatment following a vitreous haemorrhage or to treat retinal detachment, although sometimes conventional surgery may be recommended. Treatment can usually prevent deterioration in your vision but cannot restore visual loss due to retinal damage that has already occurred. If your condition stabilizes after treatment, the time between your eye examinations may gradually increase.

Cataracts

If you have diabetes, you are more prone to cataracts, in which the lens of the eye, which is normally clear, becomes cloudy. Cataracts develop as a result of changes to protein fibres in the lens. These changes are a normal part of ageing (which is why people who don't have diabetes can also develop them), but they can also be due to a blood glucose level that has been high for many years.

Symptoms and diagnosis

The cloudiness of the lens reduces the amount of light entering the eye. As a result, vision becomes blurred and distorted; in addition, bright lights may appear to have a halo. Because cataracts are progressive, they cause a gradual deterioration in vision (although not complete sight loss, as light can still enter the eye and reach the light-sensitive

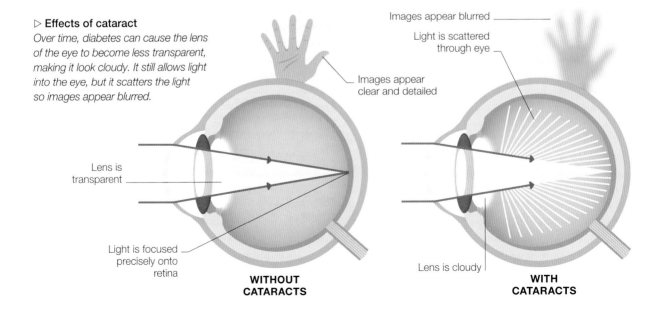

▷ **Effects of cataract**
Over time, diabetes can cause the lens of the eye to become less transparent, making it look cloudy. It still allows light into the eye, but it scatters the light so images appear blurred.

Images appear blurred

Light is scattered through eye

Images appear clear and detailed

Lens is transparent

Light is focused precisely onto retina

Lens is cloudy

WITHOUT CATARACTS

WITH CATARACTS

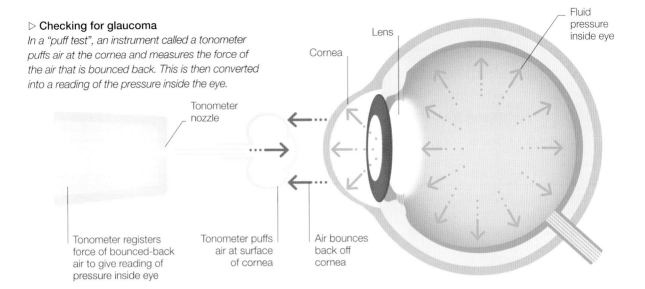

▷ **Checking for glaucoma**
*In a "puff test", an instrument called a tonometer
puffs air at the cornea and measures the force of
the air that is bounced back. This is then converted
into a reading of the pressure inside the eye.*

Cornea

Lens

Fluid
pressure
inside eye

Tonometer
nozzle

Tonometer registers
force of bounced-back
air to give reading of
pressure inside eye

Tonometer puffs
air at surface
of cornea

Air bounces
back off
cornea

retina even when cataracts are advanced). Cataracts
are diagnosed by direct inspection of the front of the
eye during an eye examination.

Prevention and treatment
You can reduce your risk of developing cataracts
by getting to, or close to, your blood glucose target
range. Cataracts develop slowly and may never reach
a stage at which they need treatment. If they seriously
impair vision, they can be surgically removed and
a new artificial lens inserted. This surgery usually
restores vision, although you will probably need
glasses or contact lenses afterwards.

Diabetes-related glaucoma
Glaucoma is a condition in which the pressure of the
fluid inside your eye becomes too high. The pressure
can damage the retina and, if untreated, can lead to
loss of vision. Glaucoma can affect anybody, but
people with diabetic retinopathy are at increased
risk of developing it. Glaucoma may not produce
noticeable symptoms in its early stages, but later it
may cause pain and increasing visual impairment.

Glaucoma can be detected during a routine eye
examination by a simple "puff test" to measure the
pressure inside the eye. It can usually be treated

successfully, either with medication or with surgery.
Treatment should prevent any further deterioration
in vision, although any vision loss that has already
occurred will be permanent.

Living with reduced vision
If your vision is adversely affected by retinopathy or
cataracts, making adjustments in your life may help
you to cope. There are various benefits and other
forms of support to help you do this. To find out
more, contact a national organization for people
with reduced vision or diabetes, or both.

Impaired vision could affect your ability to
manage daily tasks, and specifically those that are
related to your diabetes. If you find that checking
your blood glucose level, taking tablets, and/or
injecting yourself is difficult, ask your health
professional about aids that can make things easier,
for example "talking" glucose meters, large displays,
and click pen devices. Hypos (see pp.62–67) can
be problematic because you may not be able to see
well enough to treat yourself. You can ask someone
close to you for help with these tasks, or ask your
health professional for their ideas and support. If
you drive, you may need to establish whether it
is safe for you to continue driving.

Urinary system conditions

People with diabetes are at increased risk of developing problems with the urinary system – the kidneys, ureters (tubes from the kidneys to the bladder), bladder, and urethra (tube from the bladder to outside the body). Common problems include cystitis (infection of the bladder) and genital candidiasis (thrush). Kidney disease (nephropathy) is also a risk, particularly for people who have had diabetes for many years.

Cystitis

Inflammation of the bladder, known as cystitis, is typically due to a bacterial infection. It is more common in people with diabetes because a slightly raised blood glucose level and/or glucose in the urine provides a good environment for bacteria to thrive.

Cystitis is thought to occur when bacteria that normally live harmlessly on the skin or in the bowel get into the bladder through the urethra. Cystitis is more common in women than men, because their urethras are shorter than men's, making it easier for bacteria to pass into the bladder. Cystitis is not classed as a sexually transmitted infection, but having sex is one way in which bacteria can get into the urinary tract. The main symptoms of cystitis include pain when urinating; a frequent and urgent need to urinate; and pain in the lower abdomen. If you have cystitis, you can treat it yourself by taking paracetamol or ibuprofen and drinking

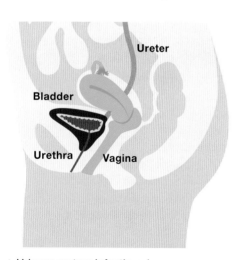

△ **Urinary system infections in women**
In women, cystitis and genital candidiasis are fairly common, even in women who do not have diabetes. Cystitis affects the bladder, whereas genital candidiasis affects the external genitals (vulva) and/or vagina.

CYSTITIS SYMPTOMS

Pain, burning, and/or stinging when urinating

Needing to urinate urgently and frequently

Pain in the lower abdomen

Dark, cloudy, or strong-smelling urine

CANDIDIASIS SYMPTOMS

Itching and irritation around the vagina

Pain, soreness, stinging when urinating or during sex

Thick, white, usually odourless discharge from the vagina

plenty of water. You should avoid sex until you feel better, as it may make the condition worse. If symptoms last for longer than three days, consult a health professional as you may need antibiotics. You should also seek advice if you are not certain your symptoms are due to cystitis.

Genital candidiasis

Commonly known as thrush, genital candidiasis is caused by a fungal infection. Like cystitis, it is more common in women than in men. It is thought to be due to overgrowth of fungi that normally live harmlessly in the body. People with diabetes are more susceptible to the condition because glucose in their urine can cause the fungi to multiply.

Candidiasis does not always cause symptoms. If they do occur, in women the main ones are itchiness and pain around the entrance of the vagina; a white discharge that may resemble

cottage cheese but does not usually smell; and pain or stinging during urination or sex. In men, there may be irritation, pain, and redness around the head of the penis and under the foreskin; a white discharge, which may resemble cottage cheese and usually smells unpleasant; and difficulty retracting the foreskin. Candidiasis is treated with an antifungal medication, available on prescription or over-the-counter.

> ↘ **AVOIDING URINARY TRACT INFECTIONS**
>
> You can reduce your risk of cystitis and candidiasis by:
>
> - Keeping your blood glucose often in your target range.
> - Drinking plenty of water.
> - Emptying your bladder frequently and completely.
> - Wearing loose cotton underwear.
> - Keeping your genitals clean, and drying fully after washing.
> - For women, wiping from front to back after a bowel movement.
> - Avoiding the use of perfumed toiletries, deodorants, or douches on your genitals.

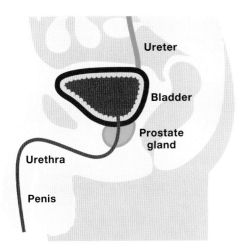

△ **Urinary system infections in men**
In men, a fungal infection may affect the head of the penis and under the foreskin, causing genital candidiasis, or bacteria may enter the urethra and move up to the prostate gland or bladder, causing cystitis.

CYSTITIS SYMPTOMS

Pain, burning, and/or stinging when urinating

Needing to urinate urgently and frequently

Pain in the lower abdomen

Dark, cloudy, or strong-smelling urine

CANDIDIASIS SYMPTOMS

Irritation, burning, and redness around the head of penis and under the foreskin

Thick, white, unpleasant-smelling discharge from the penis

Difficulty retracting the foreskin

Nephropathy

The kidneys filter the blood and remove waste products by making urine. They also regulate the amount of fluid and salts in the body, which helps to regulate blood pressure. The kidneys' main filtering units are called nephrons. Nephropathy is a general term for deterioration in the kidneys' ability to function properly, which causes illness and may lead to kidney failure.

Nephropathy that develops slowly over a period of years is known as chronic kidney disease (CKD). In this condition,

consistently raised blood glucose and blood pressure damage the nephrons. Their blood vessels become blocked, allowing protein to leak into the urine and waste products to remain in the blood.

Stages of chronic kidney disease

In the earliest stage of CKD, minute amounts of a protein called albumin are found in the urine – a condition called microalbuminuria. This does not produce any symptoms, so your health professional will carry out urine and blood tests once or twice a year to check for early signs of kidney damage.

If CKD worsens, larger amounts of protein will be found in the urine – a condition known as proteinuria. You may develop proteinuria temporarily if you have a kidney or bladder infection; the protein usually disappears when the

Glomerulus, where blood is filtered — Waste fluid

Unfiltered blood enters glomerulus

Tubule passes through net of capillaries

Unfiltered blood from renal artery

Filtered blood passing to renal vein

Capillaries reabsorb salts and water

Waste fluid enters urine-collecting duct

Unfiltered blood flows to next nephron

Filtered blood passing to renal vein

Waste leaves nephron as urine

Nephron

△ **The kidneys**
Each kidney contains about a million filtering units called nephrons. Each nephron has a glomerulus, which filters out wastes and excess fluid, and a long tubule that reabsorbs essential substances into the blood. The waste leaves the kidney as urine.

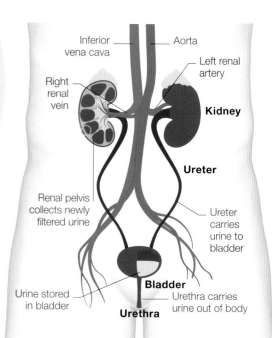

Inferior vena cava — Aorta
Right renal vein
Left renal artery
Kidney
Ureter
Renal pelvis collects newly filtered urine
Ureter carries urine to bladder
Urine stored in bladder
Bladder
Urethra carries urine out of body
Urethra

infection clears up. However, if proteinuria persists, it means the kidneys are being progressively damaged and are less able to filter out waste products or remove excess fluid from the body. Proteinuria may not always produce symptoms but losing large amounts of protein in the urine may cause problems such as swollen ankles or legs; shortness of breath; tiredness; nausea; and itchy skin. For a definite diagnosis, your health professional will carry out urine and blood tests. You may also need an ultrasound scan.

If left untreated, CKD may lead to end-stage kidney failure, in which there is permanent loss of all, or almost all, kidney function. The main symptoms of this condition include swelling of the face, limbs, and abdomen; a greatly reduced output of urine; severe lethargy; weight loss; headache; vomiting; and very itchy skin. Diagnosis and management of end-stage kidney failure will be in a specialist renal (kidney) clinic, working with your diabetes health professionals.

Prevention and treatment

Keeping your blood glucose, and particularly your blood pressure, in your target ranges is the best way to prevent CKD from developing or progressing. If microalbuminuria is diagnosed and your blood glucose is raised, you will be supported to reduce it. If you have raised blood pressure, you will be prescribed medication to lower it. Stopping smoking, losing weight if you need to, and reducing

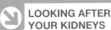

LOOKING AFTER YOUR KIDNEYS

Taking care of your kidneys is a vital part of your diabetes care; these steps can help to prevent kidney disease from developing or worsening.

- Keep your blood pressure and blood glucose within your recommended target ranges.
- Ensure your urine is tested for protein and your blood is tested for kidney function at least once a year, or more often if recommended by your health professional.
- Attend all of your medical appointments, especially your annual review.
- If you smoke, stop.
- Lose weight, if necessary.
- Try to follow healthy eating and physical activity guidelines.

salt in food will also help to lower blood pressure. You may be prescribed ACE (angiotensin-converting enzyme) inhibitor medication to help slow down the progression of CKD. Your health professionals will also monitor your blood pressure, kidney function, and blood glucose with HbA1c tests (see p.31).

If you develop proteinuria, a specialist dietitian will give you individually tailored advice, for example, about eating fewer foods that are high in potassium (such as yeast extract and bananas) or salt, to prevent wastes from building up in your body. Your diabetes medication is also likely to be changed.

If you develop end-stage kidney failure, the main treatment options are dialysis or a kidney transplant. You will also need to adjust the dose of your diabetes medication. A specialist dietitian will give personal advice about changes to your food, and you will probably also be advised to restrict your fluid intake.

Keeping your **blood glucose** and **blood pressure** well **managed** is vital to help **prevent nephropathy** from **developing** or **progressing**

Foot conditions

When you have diabetes, you are at risk of foot problems due to nerve damage in your legs (peripheral neuropathy) or poor blood circulation to your feet (peripheral ischaemia). Either or both of these conditions makes you more susceptible to associated complications, for example foot ulcers, and even severe infections, such as gangrene. However, good foot care can help prevent such problems.

Peripheral neuropathy

In peripheral neuropathy, nerves supplying your extremities (the ends of your limbs) are damaged due to repeated periods of high blood glucose, as well as high blood pressure (see pp.192–193) in the tiny vessels that supply the nerves. The damage occurs over months or years. It most commonly affects the feet, as they are supplied by the longest nerves and they bear your body weight. It may also affect the lower legs or, rarely, the arms and hands.

Symptoms and diagnosis

The main symptoms are pain and alterations in sensation (such as tingling or burning); some people don't have any symptoms, whereas in others they may be severe. The condition may come on gradually, and you may not even notice it, so your feet need to be examined by a health professional at least once a year. They will check for reddened areas caused by pressure; dry skin; calluses; wounds or open sores; abnormal warmth; and any changes in

CHARACTERISTICS OF FOOT CONDITIONS

Peripheral neuropathy and ischaemia have different characteristics. It is possible to have a combination of the conditions, known as neuroischaemia, which further increases your chances of developing foot problems.

PERIPHERAL NEUROPATHY	PERIPHERAL ISCHAEMIA
Warm skin	Cool or cold skin
Lack of feeling in foot or feet	Normal or slightly reduced feeling
May be painless, but pain can occur and is most severe at night	Painful during exertion or at rest at any time of day
Normal or increased pulses in the feet	Faint pulses in the feet, or no pulses at all
Callused skin	No calluses
Reduced reflexes	Normal reflexes
Prone to ulcers on any areas of pressure: for example, the soles of the feet	Prone to ulcers on the sides of the feet
Potential to develop Charcot (misshapen) foot	Potential to develop gangrene

the shape of your feet. To assess sensation, they will touch different areas of your feet while you have your eyes closed or are looking away, then ask you what you can feel. They will also check the reflexes in your ankles and knees, to detect any muscle weakness due to nerve damage.

Prevention, treatment, and outlook

You can reduce the likelihood of developing peripheral neuropathy by careful blood glucose management and meticulous foot care (see pp.122–123). If you do develop the condition, you will be at greater risk of damaging your feet. Your health professional will give you advice about specific risks, how to prevent them, and what to do if problems arise. You also need to check your feet daily yourself.

If the peripheral neuropathy is painful, you may be prescribed medication for pain relief. If bedding irritates your feet and legs, applying a flim dressing, or even clingfilm, may help. You can also ask your health professional about having a bed cradle to keep bedding off your feet and legs. Nerve damage that has already occurred is irreversible; however, you can stop it getting worse by careful blood glucose management and good personal foot care.

Peripheral ischaemia

In this condition, the blood supply to your legs and feet is reduced due to narrowing of the arteries, which deprives your legs and feet of oxygen and nutrients. This narrowing may be caused by atherosclerosis (build-up of fatty areas inside arteries). Factors that increase the risk of developing peripheral ischaemia include smoking, high blood cholesterol, a high-fat diet, and persistently raised blood glucose levels.

Symptoms and diagnosis

Symptoms include cramps, cold skin, and wounds that don't heal properly. As the symptoms usually develop over months or years and you may not even notice any changes, you must have your feet

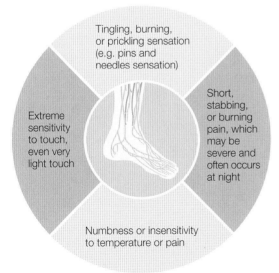

△ **Common symptoms of peripheral neuropathy**
Peripheral neuropathy may not produce noticeable symptoms, or the symptoms may change over time. Any symptoms may affect the toes, a small part of one foot, parts of both feet, or all of both feet.

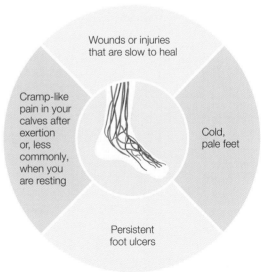

△ **Common symptoms of peripheral ischaemia**
Symptoms of peripheral ischaemia tend to develop slowly. Typically, both legs and/or feet are affected at the same time, although in some people the symptoms may be worse in one leg or foot.

▷ **Charcot foot**
Untreated, Charcot foot can lead to permanent damage to the foot bones, resulting in a misshapen foot.

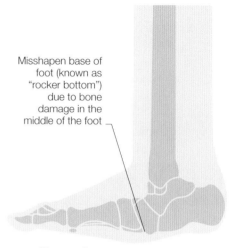

Misshapen base of foot (known as "rocker bottom") due to bone damage in the middle of the foot

Normal foot structure

Healthy foot

Charcot foot

examined by a health professional at least once a year. As well as testing your nerve responses (see p.189), they will check the pulses in your feet; a faint or absent pulse may indicate ischaemia.

Prevention, treatment, and outlook
You can help to prevent peripheral ischaemia by eating healthily; not smoking; regular physical activity; taking your medication as recommended; and careful blood glucose management.

If you are diagnosed with peripheral ischaemia, you will be referred for scans and other tests to investigate the blood flow in your legs. Peripheral ischaemia is irreversible, but it can often be stabilized or treated to improve blood flow. If the ischaemia is mild, your health professional may advise lifestyle changes and/or medication to prevent the condition from

getting worse. If it is more severe, you may be advised to have surgery to widen or bypass affected blood vessels.

Possible complications
Untreated, peripheral neuropathy or ischaemia can lead to potentially serious complications, including Charcot foot, ulcers, and possibly loss of the blood supply, which may result in gangrene.

Charcot foot
A complication of peripheral neuropathy, Charcot foot can result in permanent foot deformity. In this condition, the bones of the feet become weaker and easily damaged, so that even a minor injury can cause them to disintegrate or fracture. New bone forms at the site of the damage but the foot becomes misshapen as a result. An early sign is a hot, swollen, painful foot that gets worse over 2–3 months. To treat it, your health professional may advise you to keep weight off the foot; they may also fit you with a cast in the short term and specially made footwear in the long term.

Untreated, peripheral neuropathy and/or ischaemia can lead to potentially serious complications

ASSESSING YOUR RISK OF FOOT ULCERS

You are likely to develop foot ulcers if:

- Your blood glucose level has been above 10 mmol/L for long periods of time.
- Your blood pressure is over 140/80 and is not properly treated with medication.
- You have pins and needles or a burning sensation in your feet, or the skin there is acutely sensitive.
- You smoke.
- You have had foot ulcers before.
- You have poor circulation in your legs.
- You have reduced sensation in parts of your feet.

Foot ulcers

Ulcers may result from either neuropathy or ischaemia. They are most likely to occur on the soles of the feet or on areas subjected to pressure (for example, from tight shoes). Ulcers need immediate attention to prevent serious damage or infection. Check your feet every day. If you have any wounds, bruises, or calluses that don't start to heal after a few days, or any red, hot areas, alert your health professional as soon as you can. They will clean and dress any ulcers, give you antibiotics to treat infection, and fit you with a cast or footwear to protect the area from pressure as it heals.

Gangrene

This is a complication of peripheral ischaemia in which tissues lose their blood supply completely. The skin turns bluish-purple and then black. To prevent it, any wounds or sores must be treated as soon as possible. If a toe or foot develops gangrene, amputation may even be needed to stop the damage spreading.

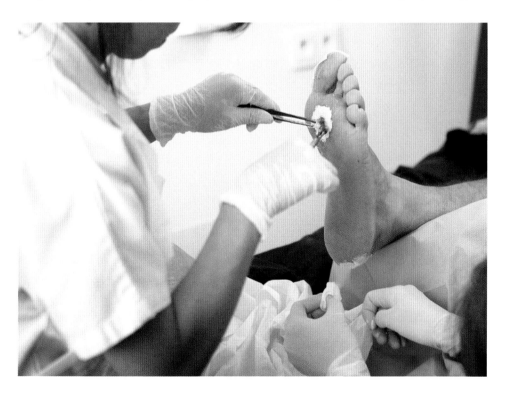

◁ **Treating a foot ulcer**
If you have a foot ulcer, your health professional will clean out the infected tissue then dress the wound to prevent further infection.

Cardiovascular conditions

Diabetes is strongly linked to high blood pressure and hyperlipidaemia (high blood lipid levels), which as well as being cardiovascular (heart and circulatory) conditions themselves, are also major risk factors for other cardiovascular problems. Identifying your risk factors and making relevant changes to your lifestyle will help to prevent heart and circulation problems from developing.

High blood pressure

Known medically as hypertension, high blood pressure is a contributor to other complications of diabetes, such as eye problems (see pp.180–183), kidney conditions (see pp.184–187), coronary heart disease (see pp.194–195), stroke (see p.196), and peripheral vascular disease (see p.197). The link between high blood pressure and diabetes is not yet fully understood, but it may be partly related to the level of insulin in the blood. In type 1 diabetes, high blood pressure also often occurs if your kidney function starts to deteriorate; in type 2 diabetes, it is linked with hyperlipidaemia and being overweight.

Being less active, smoking, high alcohol consumption, and stress are also risk factors. Addressing any or all of these can help to prevent high blood pressure (see panel, p.197).

High blood pressure rarely produces symptoms. If you have diabetes and a blood pressure of 140/80 millimetres of mercury (mmHg) or above when you are tested on several occasions, you will be diagnosed with high blood pressure. The first figure refers to the pressure when your heart contracts, the second figure refers to when your heart relaxes between beats.

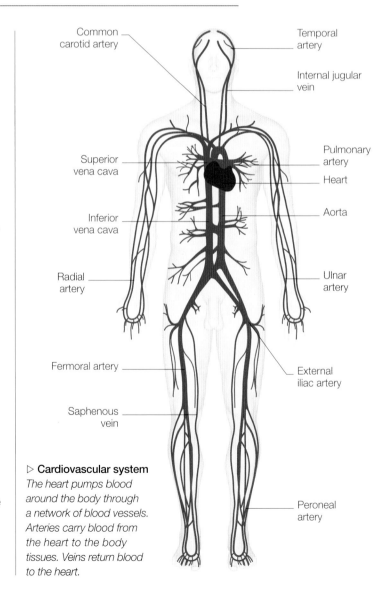

Common carotid artery · Temporal artery · Internal jugular vein · Superior vena cava · Pulmonary artery · Heart · Aorta · Inferior vena cava · Radial artery · Ulnar artery · Fermoral artery · External iliac artery · Saphenous vein · Peroneal artery

▷ **Cardiovascular system**
The heart pumps blood around the body through a network of blood vessels. Arteries carry blood from the heart to the body tissues. Veins return blood to the heart.

BLOOD LIPID LEVELS

Lipid levels are measured by analysing a blood sample for HDL (high-density lipoprotein) cholesterol, LDL (low-density lipoprotein) cholesterol, and often also for triglycerides. HDL cholesterol is often called "good" cholesterol, because it helps to lower blood levels of LDL ("bad") cholesterol. Triglycerides are carried in the blood and used for energy or stored as body fat. In general, the goal is to have a low total lipid level, a low level of LDL cholesterol, a low level of triglycerides, and a relatively high level of HDL cholesterol.

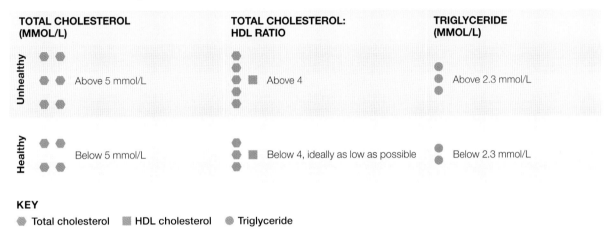

TOTAL CHOLESTEROL (MMOL/L)	TOTAL CHOLESTEROL: HDL RATIO	TRIGLYCERIDE (MMOL/L)
Unhealthy — Above 5 mmol/L	Above 4	Above 2.3 mmol/L
Healthy — Below 5 mmol/L	Below 4, ideally as low as possible	Below 2.3 mmol/L

KEY
Total cholesterol   HDL cholesterol   Triglyceride

If you are diagnosed with high blood pressure, you will be prescribed medication to lower it, and your blood pressure will be reviewed every three to six months. It may be necessary to take more than one type of medication, but treatment is usually very effective.

Hyperlipidaemia

A high level of lipids (fats and fat-like substances, such as cholesterol) in the blood, referred to as hyperlipidaemia, is a major cause of coronary heart disease, stroke, and peripheral artery disease. It is more common in people with type 2 diabetes. The link between diabetes and hyperlipidaemia is not fully understood, but in type 2 diabetes, the high level of insulin caused by insulin resistance is thought to be partly responsible. If you have type 2 diabetes, you are more likely to develop hyperlipidaemia if you are overweight and have high blood pressure. Other general risk factors in either type 1 or type 2 diabetes include eating foods high in saturated fats, inactivity, smoking, an underactive thyroid gland, and a raised blood glucose level over years. A high alcohol intake and/or family history of hyperlipidaemia are also risk factors. In general, your likelihood of developing hyperlipidaemia can be reduced by self-care measures (see panel, p.197).

Hyperlipidaemia rarely produces symptoms. At your annual review (see pp.142–143) you will be offered a blood test to measure your lipid levels. If your levels are outside the healthy range, you will be offered advice and possibly also medication, such as statins, to reduce your lipid levels. Subsequently, your blood lipid levels may be checked every 3–6 months to assess how well the treatment is working.

Having **diabetes** means you are at increased **risk** of developing **coronary heart disease**

Coronary heart disease

In coronary heart disease (CHD), fatty deposits known as atheromas (also sometimes called plaques) build up in the coronary arteries – the two main arteries that supply the heart itself with blood – and restrict blood flow to the heart muscle.

Having diabetes means that you are at increased risk of developing CHD. Other risk factors include high blood pressure, hyperlipidaemia, a high intake of saturated fat, lack of physical activity, smoking, being overweight, a family history of CHD, and a blood glucose level that has been persistently raised for a period of years. Taking steps to reduce any of these risk factors will help you to avoid CHD (see panel, p.197).

When blood flow through the coronary arteries is restricted, you may experience angina, a heart attack, or heart failure.

● **Angina** This produces a temporary sensation of pain or pressure in your chest. You may also experience pain in your left shoulder or down the inner side of your left arm, especially when you are stressed or exert yourself.

● **Heart attack** This typically causes severe pain in the centre of your chest that may spread to the jaw, neck, arms, or back; breathlessness, palpitations, sweating, lightheadedness, nausea, and sometimes loss of consciousness. However, some people have very mild or no symptoms. A severe heart attack may be rapidly life-threatening.

● **Heart failure** In this condition, the heart becomes less effective at pumping blood around the body. Signs of heart failure include swelling in your legs, feet, and abdomen, shortness of breath, tiredness, and lack of energy. In many people, the condition worsens slowly over time.

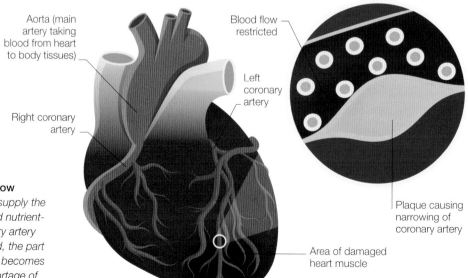

Aorta (main artery taking blood from heart to body tissues)

Right coronary artery

Blood flow restricted

Left coronary artery

Plaque causing narrowing of coronary artery

Area of damaged heart muscle

▷ **Restricted blood flow**
The coronary arteries supply the heart with oxygen- and nutrient-rich blood. If a coronary artery is narrowed or blocked, the part of the heart it supplies becomes damaged due to a shortage of oxygen and nutrients.

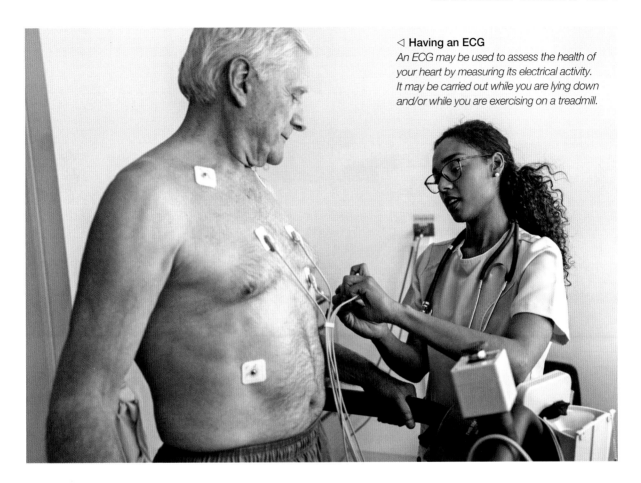

◁ **Having an ECG**
An ECG may be used to assess the health of your heart by measuring its electrical activity. It may be carried out while you are lying down and/or while you are exercising on a treadmill.

CHD may be diagnosed by means of an electrocardiogram (ECG) in which the heart's electrical impulses are recorded. Various imaging techniques may also be used to view the heart and assess the health of the coronary arteries.

CHD may be treated with medication, surgery, or a combination of both. If you have a heart attack and are admitted to hospital, your diabetes will be treated with an insulin infusion, possibly followed by insulin injections at home for several months afterwards. You may or may not need to keep using insulin in the longer term, depending on your blood glucose levels and other risk factors.

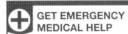 **GET EMERGENCY MEDICAL HELP**

If you have symptoms of a heart attack:

- Intense pain in the centre of your chest that may spread to your jaw, neck, arms, or back, shortness of breath, weakness and/or lightheadedness, sweating, nausea, and sometimes loss of consciousness.

If you have symptoms of a stroke:

- Facial weakness, which may cause drooping of your face, mouth, or eye on one side, drooling, and loss of your ability to smile; weakness or numbness in your arms; problems speaking, such as slurred or garbled speech; and/or confusion and disorientation.

Stroke

A stroke is an interruption to the blood supply to the brain, causing brain cells to be damaged or destroyed. There are two main types of stroke: an ischaemic stroke, due to blockage of a blood vessel, and a haemorrhagic stroke, caused by a burst blood vessel.

There are two main risk factors for stroke: high blood pressure and atherosclerosis, both of which are more common in people with diabetes. In atherosclerosis, fatty deposits build up inside the arteries and narrow them; a clot may then block the artery. When this happens in an artery that supplies the brain, a stroke occurs. Careful blood glucose management and applying good health principles can reduce your risk of having a stroke (see panel, opposite).

Paying attention to your diabetes and general health can help to reduce your risk of a stroke

The symptoms of a stroke vary according to which part of the brain has been damaged. Movement, speech, memory, vision, hearing, or balance may be affected. Typically, however, symptoms include facial weakness, which may cause drooping of one side of the face, drooping of the mouth, and loss of the ability to smile; weakness or numbness of one or both arms; and speech problems, such as slurred or garbled speech or even a complete inability to speak. A severe stroke may cause unconsciousness and coma, which may be life-threatening.

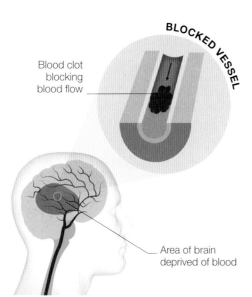

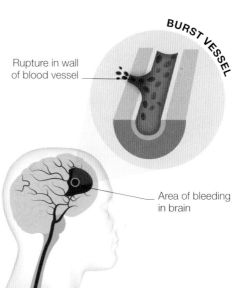

△ **Ischaemic stroke**
An ischaemic stroke is due to blockage of a blood vessel by a clot, formed either in the vessel itself or carried there from elsewhere in the body. Blood cannot reach part of the brain and brain tissue is damaged as a result.

△ **Haemorrhagic stroke**
A haemorrhagic stroke occurs as a result of a ruptured blood vessel and subsequent bleeding on the surface of the brain or within the brain. The blood that accumulates presses on the brain, damaging brain tissue.

A stroke is diagnosed from your symptoms and/or a brain scan. The immediate treatment varies according to the type of stroke but may include medication and/or surgery. Longer-term treatment typically includes rehabilitation therapies, such as physiotherapy or speech therapy. Some people make a good recovery, but others are left with long-term problems.

Peripheral vascular disease

In peripheral vascular disease (PVD), fatty deposits (known as atheromas or plaques) in the arteries of the legs or, less commonly, the arms and restrict blood flow. Without treament, PVD may lead to a condition known as peripheral ischaemia, in which blood flow to the extremities is severely reduced. This, in turn, may lead to serious complications, such as gangrene (see pp.188-191).

Various factors increase your risk of developing PVD, including a high level of insulin in the blood; a blood glucose level that has been consistently raised for a period of years; high blood pressure (see p.192); and hyperlipidaemia (see p.193). Being less active, smoking, and being overweight also increase your risk.

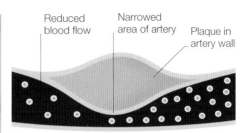

Artery

△ **Narrowing of peripheral arteries**
In peripheral vascular disease, fatty plaques in the walls of arteries in the legs and/or arms reduce blood flow, leading to symptoms such as muscle pain and fatigue.

As well as personal action to reduce your risk (see panel, below), it is also important to have your blood pressure and blood lipid levels monitored regularly, and take any necessary treatment for these conditions.

The main sign of PVD is pain and fatigue in the leg or arm muscles during physical activity; typically, the greater the exertion, the greater the pain. PVD is diagnosed from your symptoms and medical history, together with imaging of your arms and/or legs. Treatment is with medication, and sometimes surgery to widen, bypass, or replace affected areas of artery.

**REDUCING YOUR RISK OF
CARDIOVASCULAR CONDITIONS**

The risk of developing cardiovascular problems can be significantly reduced by various health-related measures you can do yourself:

- Eat healthily. Include plenty of fruit and vegetables, and limit the amount of saturated fat and salt in your food.
- Be as physically active as possible.
- Stop smoking.
- If you are overweight, try to lose excess weight (see pp.94–99).

- Pay attention to your diabetes management.
- Drink alcohol within recommended limits.
- Take any medication you have been prescribed to reduce your blood pressure and/or blood lipid levels. If you experience any side effects, report them promptly.
- Try to minimize the effects of stress (see p.111).

Other conditions

If you have had diabetes for a long time, you are at risk of developing a number of conditions, such as skin problems at injection sites; dental problems; sexual problems; and problems with nerves controlling automatic body functions (known as autonomic neuropathy). The chance of developing these problems can be reduced by careful blood glucose management and a healthy lifestyle.

Lipohypertrophy

Lumpy skin tissue at injection sites is known as lipohypertrophy. The lumps are swollen and raised, but not red or painful. They are due to repeated injections at the same site causing fat deposits to build up under the skin. Insulin itself can also cause overgrowth of tissues where the skin has been damaged by injections.

The lumps usually develop slowly, so you may not notice anything wrong. Run your hand across your injection sites to check whether the skin feels different there. If you cannot feel any lumps but your blood glucose fluctuates from day to day for no apparent reason, talk to your health professional. Unpredictable swings in your blood glucose indicate that you may be injecting into sites where the tissue under the skin is abnormal (even though there may be no visible sign of this) and this may be affecting insulin absorption. Your health professional will be able to tell you if you have lipohypertrophy or areas of abnormal skin tissue by examining your injection sites.

To avoid lipohypertrophy, rotate your injection sites (see p.56) and change your needle as recommended. If you already have lipohypertrophy, avoid injecting in the affected areas. If insulin absorption has been a problem, you may need to reduce your insulin dose when you use a new injection site; your health professional will be able to advise. Over time, the lumps should gradually get smaller.

Insulin pen

Fatty lump

Needle

Subcutaneous fatty tissue

Outer layer of skin

◁ **Lumpy skin**
Damage from repeated injections at the same site, together with the effects of insulin, may cause fatty lumps (lipohypertrophy) to develop under the skin.

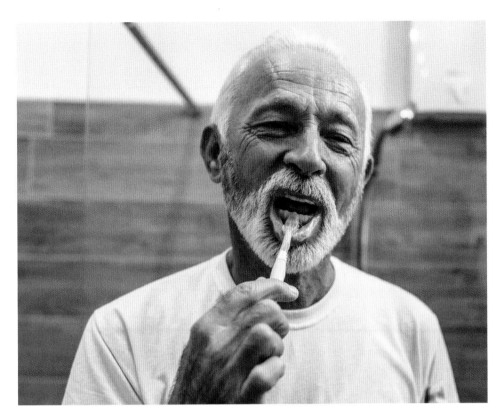

◁ **Oral hygiene**
Daily care of your teeth by brushing and using floss or interdental brushes to clean between your teeth can prevent the build-up of plaque and bacteria and reduce the risk of tooth decay and gum disease.

Dental problems

Diabetes carries a risk of developing various dental problems, including gum disease, tooth decay (dental caries), and mouth infections. This is mainly because raised blood glucose can lead to more glucose in the saliva, which provides a good environment for bacteria to thrive in the mouth. The bacteria produce acid, which attacks the teeth and can also lead to gum damage.

The main early indications of dental problems include abnormal redness and/or soreness of your gums, sensitive or painful teeth, and bad breath. If you experience any of these, see your dentist to get early treatment and help prevent any future problems from developing, such as a severe gum infection, loss of teeth, or both.

Rotating injection sites can reduce the risk of developing lumps at those sites

KEEPING YOUR MOUTH HEALTHY

You can help avoid mouth and tooth problems from developing by following good dental hygiene and careful diabetes management.

- Monitor your blood glucose regularly and try to keep the level within your target range.
- Brush your teeth at least twice a day to minimize plaque build-up.
- Clean between your teeth with floss or interdental brushes to help keep your gums healthy.
- Use a fluoride toothpaste.
- Have regular dental check-ups.
- Do not smoke.
- Try to eat food that is low in sugar. Include a variety of fresh fruit and vegetables containing vitamin C, which is essential for gum health.
- If you wear dentures, make sure you clean them frequently.

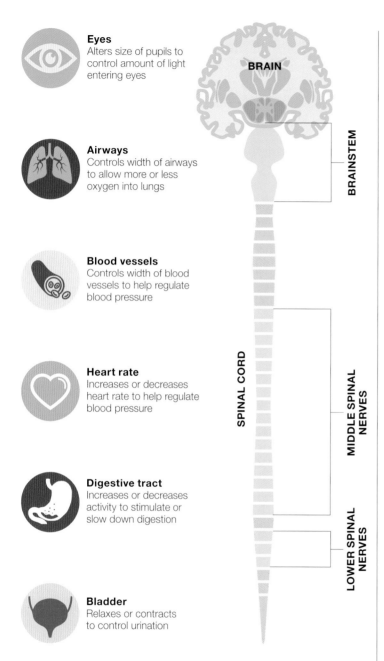

Eyes
Alters size of pupils to control amount of light entering eyes

Airways
Controls width of airways to allow more or less oxygen into lungs

Blood vessels
Controls width of blood vessels to help regulate blood pressure

Heart rate
Increases or decreases heart rate to help regulate blood pressure

Digestive tract
Increases or decreases activity to stimulate or slow down digestion

Bladder
Relaxes or contracts to control urination

BRAIN

BRAINSTEM

SPINAL CORD

MIDDLE SPINAL NERVES

LOWER SPINAL NERVES

△ **The autonomic nervous system**
Consisting of nerves coming from your brainstem (at the base of the brain) and the middle and lower parts of the spinal cord, the autonomic nervous system (ANS) automatically controls many basic body functions of the body, such as your heart rate and the activity of your digestive system.

Autonomic neuropathy

The autonomic nerves are those that control parts of your body which you do not move or control voluntarily. They help the body function by regulating your temperature, heart rate, and digestive system, for example. Damage to these nerves is known as autonomic neuropathy, and it can occur through longstanding diabetes or as a result of consistently raised blood glucose over many years. Autonomic neuropathy can produce a range of symptoms, including:

● Too much or too little sweating.
● Nausea, vomiting, diarrhoea, or constipation.
● Dizziness (postural hypotension) when you stand up or get out of bed.
● Difficulty exercising because your heart rate does not speed up enough to compensate for increased activity.
● Being unable to empty your bladder completely.
● Erectile dysfunction.
● Reduced awareness of hypos.

If you develop symptoms of autonomic neuropathy or if it is suspected at your annual review, your health professional will arrange for various tests to make a definite diagnosis.

You can help to prevent autonomic neuropathy by keeping your blood glucose within your recommended range. If you already have it, specific symptoms are treated as they occur. For example, you may be prescribed medication to lower blood pressure. Nerve damage that has already occurred cannot be reversed but you can reduce the likelihood of the condition progressing by careful blood glucose management, not smoking, eating healthily, and being as active as you can.

AVOIDING POSTURAL HYPOTENSION

There are various measures you can take that may help with postural hypotension.

- When you wake up, sit on the edge of the bed for a few minutes before standing up.
- Get up slowly from sitting to standing.
- Try keeping your head and shoulders raised while you sleep.
- Increase the amount of water you drink.
- Avoid sitting or standing still for long periods.
- Ask your health professional whether wearing supprt stockings at night would help.

Sexual problems

Having diabetes or raised blood glucose for many years can sometimes lead to sexual problems, such as vaginal dryness in women, which can make sex painful or erectile dysfunction (ED) in men. Also sometimes known as impotence, ED is an inability to achieve or sustain an erection. It can be caused by damage to the blood vessels and nerves that supply the penis. There are also many other causes of ED, including certain hormone disorders, side effects of some medications, stress, relationship difficulties, and depression. Your risk of ED is also increased by smoking and alcohol.

Your ED is less likely to be diabetes-related if you have erections at night or in the mornings, if your ED has developed suddenly, or if you only suffer from ED in specific situations, such as when you feel stressed. It is more likely to be linked to your diabetes if you are unable to achieve an erection at all and the problem has developed gradually. If you have repeated episodes of ED, talk with your health professional for a definite diagnosis.

Initial treatment of ED involves identifying and dealing with any underlying cause. Keeping your blood glucose within your target range is very important. Reducing your alcohol intake and stopping smoking will also help. If these measures do not restore full sexual function, you may be offered various treatments, including medication; physical treatments, such as a vacuum pump; or a talking therapy, such as cognitive behavioural therapy (see p.177). If you choose not to have treatment, ED will not adversely affect any other aspect of your diabetes nor your overall health.

▽ **Regular exercise**
Physical exercise not only helps with any circulatory problems but can also help you to control your weight and reduce stress, all of which may be contributory factors in erectile dysfunction.

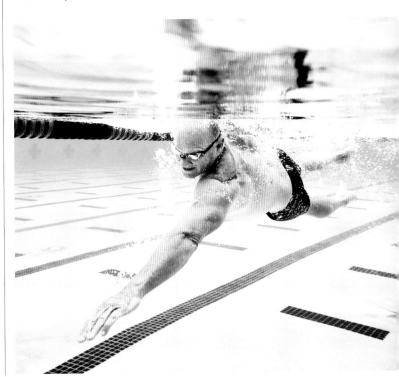

Notes

Some aspects of living with diabetes or the care recommended or available vary according to where you live. Most of the information in this book is applicable wherever you are. However, where important aspects may vary, the relevant pages or pieces of text are marked with asterisks. These direct you here, where you can find sources of information for your locality.

PREVENTING AND REVERSING DIABETES

UK
NHS education programmes are available in some areas to help prevent diabetes or put it into remission. Your diabetes health professional will be able to tell you if one is available in your area.

Australia
Individual states run prevention programmes. Contact the National Diabetes Services Scheme (NDSS; website: www.ndss.com.au) for information about the programmes in your state.

New Zealand
There are no specific prevention or reversal programmes but the Diabetes New Zealand website (www.diabetes.org.nz) gives useful self-care information.

South Africa
There are no specific prevention or reversal programmes but general information about healthy eating can be found on the Diabetes South Africa website (www.diabetessa.org.za) and on the website of the Association for Dietetics in South Africa (www.adsa.org.za).

HEALTHY EATING

UK
The dietary recommendations here are the official UK government ones. More detailed information can be found on the NHS website (www.nhs.uk/live-well/eat-well/).

Australia
The official healthy eating guidelines can be found on the government website (www.eatforhealth.gov.au)

New Zealand
The official healthy eating guidelines can be found on the government website (www.health.govt.nz)

South Africa
The recommended healthy eating guidelines can be found on the website of the Association for Dietetics in South Africa (www.adsa.org.za). The Diabetes South Africa website (www.diabetessa.org.za) also has information about healthy eating.

WORK

UK
The information on these pages applies to the UK. Additional information can be found on the Diabetes UK website (www.diabetes.org.uk).

Australia
Information about working when you have diabetes can be found on the Diabetes Australia website (www.diabetesaustralia.com.au).

New Zealand
Information about working when you have diabetes can be found on the Diabetes New Zealand website (www.diabetes.org.nz).

South Africa
Information about working when you have diabetes can be found on the Diabetes South Africa website (www.diabetessa.org.za).

DRIVING

UK
You must inform the Driver and Vehicle Licensing Agency (DVLA) if your diabetes requires insulin treatment. The DVLA can be contacted through the central government website (www.gov.uk).

Australia
You must inform the Driver Licensing Authorities in your state or territory, each of which has its own driver licensing authority website. Information about driving when you have diabetes can also be found on the National Diabetes Services Scheme website (www.ndss.com.au).

New Zealand
You must inform the New Zealand Transport Agency (NZTA; website: www.nzta.govt.nz).

South Africa
There are no official regulations concerning driving and diabetes. The Diabetes South Africa website (www.diabetessa.org.za) gives information about driving safely.

KEEPING HEALTHY

UK
Information about health screening available on the NHS can be found on the NHS website (www.nhs.uk). This website also provides information about eye tests, dental check-ups, and vaccinations.

Australia
Information about health screening is on the Department of Health website (www.health.gov.au), which also gives information about eye health, dental health, and vaccinations. The National Diabetes Services Scheme (NDSS) website (www.ndss.com.au) also has information about keeping healthy.

New Zealand
Information about health screening iis on the Ministry of Health website (www.health.govt.nz), which also provides information about dental health and vaccinations.

South Africa
Information about routine vaccinations is on the government website (www.gov.za) and is also published by the University of Cape Town on the webpage www.paediatrics.uct.ac.za

PREGNANCY

UK
The information on antenatal tests applies to the UK. More information can be found on the NHS website (www.nhs.uk).

Australia
Information about antenatal tests is on the Australian parenting website (www.raisingchildren.net.au).

New Zealand
Information about antenatal tests is on the Ministry of Health website (www.health.govt.nz).

South Africa
Information about antenatal tests is on the Department of Health website (www.health.gov.za).

BENEFITING FROM HEALTH CARE

UK

The health checks for people with diabetes that are described on these pages are the usual ones for adults in the UK. More information can be found on the website of Diabetes UK (www.diabetes.org.uk).

Australia

Information about health checks for people who have diabetes can be found on the National Diabetes Services Scheme (NDSS) website (www.ndss.com.au).

New Zealand

Information about health checks for people with diabetes is on the Diabetes New Zealand website (www.diabetes.org.nz).

South Africa

Information about health checks for people with diabetes is on the Diabetes South Africa website (www.diabetessa.org.za)

TEENAGERS AND YOUNG ADULTS: GETTING ON WITH YOUR LIFE

UK

The diabetes care for teenagers and young adults outlined on this page applies to the UK.

More information can be found on the website of Diabetes UK (www.diabetes.org.uk).

Australia

Information about diabetes care for teenagers and young adults can be found on the National Diabetes Services Scheme (NDSS) website (www.ndss.com.au).

New Zealand

Information about diabetes care and support for teenagers can be found on the Diabetes New Zealand website (www.diabetes.org.nz).

South Africa

Information about diabetes care for teenagers can be found on the Diabetes South Africa website (www.diabetes.org.za) and on the Youth with Diabetes website (www.youthwithdiabetes.com).

Useful resources

The organizations listed below provide useful additional information for people living with diabetes. Many also offer links to sources of emotional support and can help you to make contact with other people who live with diabetes. Your health professional is also an important source of additional information.

UK-BASED

Diabetes UK
www.diabetes.org.uk

National Institute for Health and Clinical Excellence (NICE)
www.nice.org.uk/guidance/conditions-and-diseases/diabetes-and-other-endocrinal--nutritional-and-metabolic-conditions/diabetes

NHS England Diabetes
www.england.nhs.uk/diabetes

NHS England Type 2 Diabetes Prevention Programme
www.england.nhs.uk/diabetes/diabetes-prevention

NHS Wales Diabetes
www.wales.nhs.uk/healthtopics/conditions/diabetes

NHS Scotland interactive diabetes website
www.mydiabetesmyway.scot.nhs.uk

Diabetes Network for Northern Ireland
www.hscboard.hscni.net/diabetes-network/

Juvenile Diabetes Research Foundation (UK)
www.jdrf.org.uk

Mental Health Foundation
www.mental health.org.uk

Successful Diabetes
www.successfuldiabetes.com

Type 1 Diabetes UK Immunotherapy Consortium
www.type1diabetesresearch.org.uk

Type 1 Resources (T1 Resources)
www.t1resources.uk

UK Diabetes Online Community Twitter account
@thegbdoc
Discussion forum: #gbdoc

Carbs and Cals
www.carbsandcals.com

OTHER RESOURCES

World Health Organization Diabetes
www.who.int/health-topics/diabetes#tab=tab

Diabetes Ireland
www.diabetes.ie

American Diabetes Association
www.diabetes.org

Juvenile Diabetes Research Foundation (US)
www.jdrf.org

Diabetes Canada
www.diabetes.ca

Diabetes Australia
www.diabetesaustralia.com.au

National Diabetes Services Scheme (Australia)
www.ndss.com.au

Diabetes New Zealand
www.diabetes.org.nz

Diabetes South Africa
www.diabetessa.org.za

Index

Page numbers in **bold** refer to a main entry. Page numbers in *italics* refer to illustrations.

Acknowledgments

Author's acknowledgments
I would like to thank the DK editors, designers, and wider production team for guiding me through the publication process. Also, and especially, all those people with diabetes, diabetes professionals, friends, and family who have inspired me, helped with queries, and given me support and encouragement whilst writing this book. In addition, I would like to express my appreciation to Judith Carpenter, Alan Hallett, Lisa Miner, Karen Richardson, and Jackie Sturt for their specific contributions.

Publisher's acknowledgments
DK would like to thank the following people for their help in the preparation of this book: Katie John for additional editorial help; Jemima Dunne for proofreading; and Gillian Northcott Liles for the index.

DK India would like to thank Aarushi Dhawan and Nobina Chakravorty for design assistance; Aashirwad Jain for editorial assistance; and Rakesh Kumar (DTP Designer), Priyanka Sharma (Jackets Editorial Coordinator), and Saloni Singh (Managing Jackets Editor).

Rosemary, or Rosie, Walker, RN, BSc (Hons), MA (Education)
Rosie is a former NHS diabetes specialist nurse who has also often contributed to national developments in diabetes care. She runs Successful Diabetes, a company providing education, resources and consultancy for people living or working with diabetes. In her work, she is particularly concerned to highlight and support the emotional as well as physical aspects of living with diabetes. Her full biography can be found at www.successfuldiabetes.com